Why We Walk

The Inspirational Journey Toward
a Cure *for* Breast Cancer

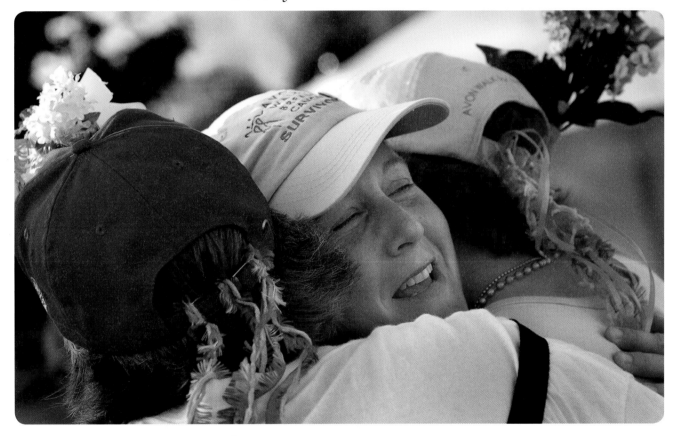

EDITED BY DEB MURPHY *with* PHOTOGRAPHS BY PAULA LERNER

TEXT BY JOHN YOW

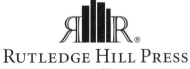

RUTLEDGE HILL PRESS
NASHVILLE, TENNESSEE
A Division of Thomas Nelson Publishers
Since 1798

www.thomasnelson.com

Published by Rutledge Hill Press, a division of Thomas Nelson, Inc., P.O. Box 141000, Nashville, Tennessee 37214.

Rutledge Hill Press books may be purchased in bulk for educational, business, fundraising, or sales promotional use.
For information, please e-mail SpecialMarkets@ThomasNelson.com.

Design: Carley Wilson Brown

Library of Congress Cataloging-in-Publication Data
Yow, John.
    Why we walk : the inspirational journey toward a cure for breast cancer /
edited by Deb Murphy ; with photographs by Paula Lerner ; text by John Yow.
        p. cm.
    ISBN 1-4016-0220-7 (hardcover)
    1. Breast—Cancer. 2. Breast—Cancer—Patients—United States—Biography.
3. Walk-a-thons—United States. I. Murphy, Debra Marie. II. Lerner, Paula. III. Title.
RC280.B8Y69 2005
362.196'99449'00922—dc22   2005009986

Printed in the United States of America
05 06 07 08 09 — 5 4 3 2 1

Contents

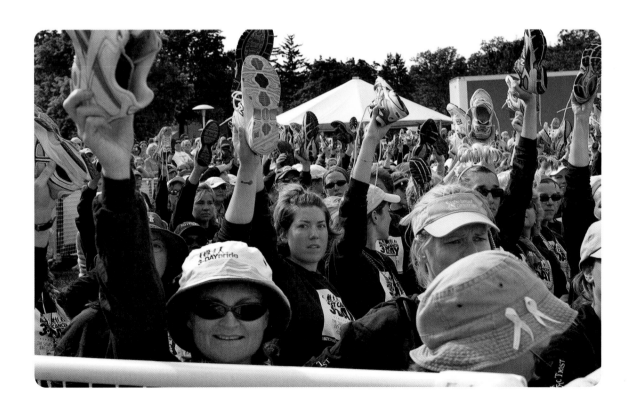

One of the most remarkable things that happened

while working on *Why We Walk* is that songwriters Phil and Julie Vassar

heard about the book and were inspired to write a moving song about ordinary individuals

united in an extraordinary purpose: to find a cure in the fight against breast cancer.

Julie Vassar tells the story of how the song came to be. *—Deb Murphy*

On a recent flight from New York City to Nashville, I had the pleasure of meeting a gentleman named David Dunham, Senior Vice President and Group Publisher at Thomas Nelson Publishers. As fate would have it, we discovered that our lives were strangely connected. Rutledge Hill Press, one of Nelson's book imprints, had recently released a CD book called *This Is God* written by my husband, Phil. David was excited to share the news of a unique project in the works called *Why We Walk* and mentioned that it would be wonderful to include an original song along with the text. After Phil and I read the gripping and heartfelt stories of people who have been devastated by breast cancer yet maintain hope through walking for a cure, we felt overwhelmingly compelled to write a song in their honor. We are humbled and privileged to be a part of this special publication and pray that others will find a sense of hope and promise in the lyric.

—Julie Vassar

Why We Walk

Music and lyrics by Phil and Julie Vassar

There's an empty seat at the dinner table
Where a mother used to sit.
She was 34 years old, full of life and dreams
And two small kids.
There's a young man with a tear in his eye and a pink ribbon on his coat
In memory of the only love he'd ever known.

There's a lady looking in the mirror without a single strand of hair.
She barely recognizes the woman standing there.
She's waging a silent war against an enemy inside
And putting up the fight of her life.

That's why we walk.
We walk to remember.
We walk to celebrate.
That's why we walk.
Leaning on each other
And holding on to faith.
For those who are gone and those who live on.
We honor them all
And that's why we walk.

She lays in a cold white room in a baby-blue paper gown,
Anticipating what the X-rays might have found.
Then she hears the words that always stop you on a dime
And prays that they found it in time.

That's why we walk.
We walk to remember.
We walk to celebrate.
That's why we walk.
Leaning on each other
And holding on to faith.
For those who are gone and those who live on.
We honor them all
And that's why we walk.

For life, for love, for one another,
For him, for her, there's strength in numbers.

Behind the Breast Cancer Walks

"It's wonderful to know that every dollar we raise brings us one step closer to a cure." —Anne Thorsen, American Cancer Society, Director of Special Events, Long Island, New York

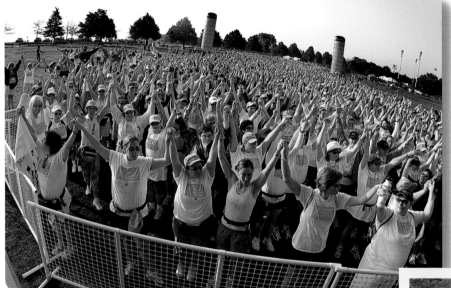

Because they were breast cancer survivors, or dear friends or relatives of those who had lost the fight against breast cancer, or those still fighting the disease, and they had had enough.

Here's what happened. These thousands of women and men, with their blistered feet and cramping muscles and popping bladders and sunscreen-slathered faces, had the time of their lives. They laughed, they sang silly songs, they hugged, they told their stories, they cried, and they forged a community that has become an unstoppable force in the ongoing battle to find a cure for this devastating disease.

W hat has become an incredible national phenomenon began in 1998, when Avon, as part of its worldwide Breast Cancer Crusade, put together the first series of three-day, 60-mile walks in support of the battle to end breast cancer. There must have been some raised eyebrows around the conference table when the concept was first proposed, but—*lo and behold!*—it turns out that thousands of women and men were more than ready to wear blisters on their aching feet by walking 20 miles a day, to submit to the indignity of porta-potties, to collapse, bone-weary, on the ground at night in little two-person tents, and to get up the next day and do it all over again. Why?

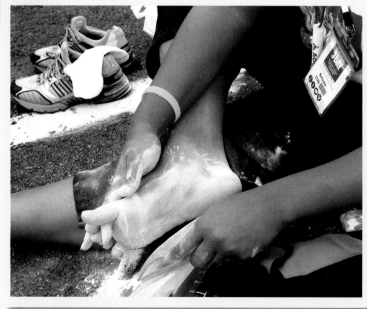

In 2003, the Breast Cancer 3-Day came under the aegis of the Susan G. Komen Breast Cancer Foundation, in partnership with the National Philanthropic Trust. (No stranger to breast cancer participatory events, the Komen Foundation has for 20 years sponsored the largest series of 5K runs/fitness walks in the world, which, with its appeal to walkers of all ages, attracts more than 1 million participants each year.)

That same year, 2003, the Avon Foundation created the Avon Walk for Breast Cancer, a weekend long-distance walk where participants sign up to walk a full marathon (26.2 miles) on Saturday, followed by a half-marathon (13.1 miles) on Sunday. These two series—the Breast Cancer 3-Day and the Avon Walk for Breast Cancer—both of which now hold multiple events each year, are the source for most of the stories that follow.

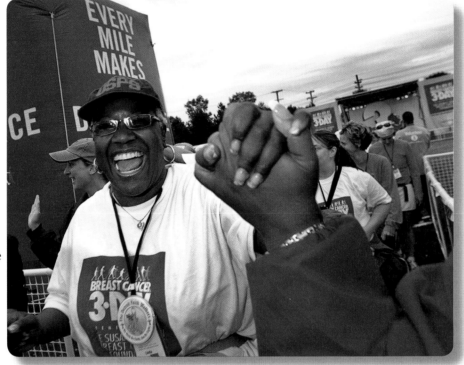

The two events have much in common—most significantly, their common purpose, their huge popularity, and their tremendous effectiveness.

In addition, both require what would seem to be a formidable commitment—of time, muscle power, and money. To participate in the Breast Cancer 3-Day, walkers pledge to raise $2,100; for the Avon Walk, the amount is $1,800. Though many walkers profess to have been at first intimidated by the prospect of "asking people for money," those same walkers often end up surprised by how easy their fundraising turns out to be. In many cases, they find that the generosity springs from the fact that more people have been touched by breast cancer than they ever would have expected. Still, for those daunted by the fundraising task, both organizations stand by to offer expert advice and creative ideas. And, in fact, the average amount raised per walker far exceeds the minimum required.

As for the time commitment, in the case of both events, the actual walks themselves are just the beginning—or, more accurately, just the ending. Whether you're walking 60 miles or 39.3, you are advised to train in advance, and both organizations offer training tips and schedules and volunteer-run training walks to help walkers shape up over the months leading up to the event. Both also strongly recommend (and offer help with) the formation of teams, both for training and for participation in the walk. Several are featured in the pages that follow, and members of teams like the Detroit Faith Walkers or Peggy's Spirit will all agree on one thing: those 10-mile training walks on early Saturday mornings are a lot easier to face in the company of others devoted to the cause.

Still, there's no disguising the fact that both events are physically demanding, and for those who want to be a part of the cause but who aren't sure they can handle the long hike, both organizations offer two other ways to participate: as crew members or as volunteers. Crew members commit to the entire walk weekend, including the Friday- and/or Saturday-night sleepovers, and perform a wide variety of tasks essential to making the event successful, including marking the route, picking up trash, setting up

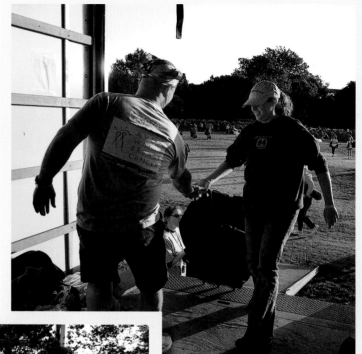

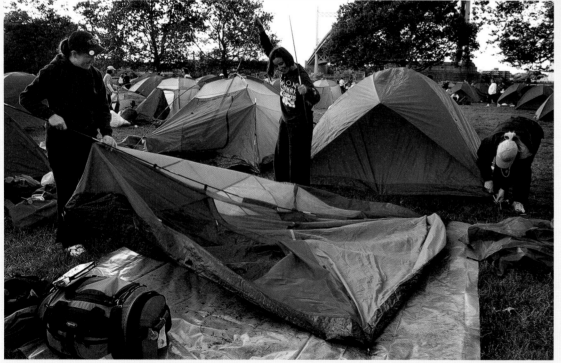

rest stops, pouring water, and everything in between. Volunteers work shorter shifts, including some in advance of the event, depending on how much time they can commit, and their jobs vary throughout the weekend to cover wherever support is most needed.

Both crew members and volunteers will testify that the most rewarding role they play is that of cheerleader, and walkers agree that the

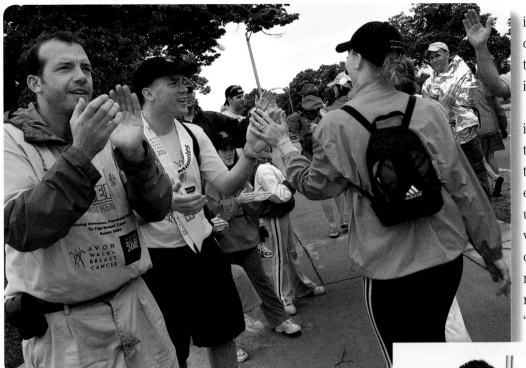

importance of the community they are creating—the sharing, the bonding, the empowerment that are so crucial in the battle against breast cancer.

The walkers themselves understand it even better. Though they're sometimes at a loss for words to describe the full impact and meaning of the walk experience, one phrase they frequently use is *life changing*. Time and again walkers characterize the world of the cancer walk—with its sense of communal purpose, of fellowship, and camaraderie, with its laughter and tears—as "how the world should be every day."

enthusiastic encouragement they receive from the folks like "Pretty Woman Man" or Paul Boulanger and Men with Heart makes all the difference in the world to their tired bodies and sometimes flagging spirits. In fact, many walkers return to the event as crew members or volunteers just to experience the event from both perspectives, and many crew members and volunteers return as walkers.

Perhaps most critically, the essence of both events is the "weekend experience." Whether it's the two nights "in camp" at the Breast Cancer 3-Day or the one night in the Wellness Village at the Avon Walk, both organizations highlight the value of keeping the walkers together for the duration of the event, up to and including the always moving closing ceremonies. Both groups understand the

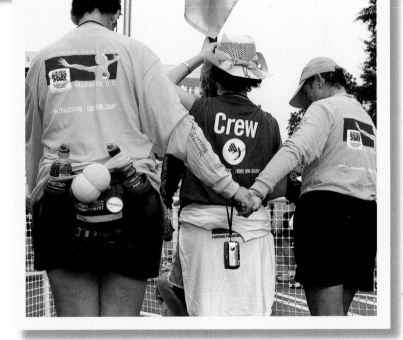

As for their record of success, the Komen Foundation–NPT partnership put on 10 events in 2004, which attracted approximately 18,000 participants and raised 26 million dollars to support breast cancer research, education, screening, and treatment programs. The 14 Avon Walk for Breast Cancer events in 2003–2004 gathered some 23,000 participants and raised approximately $60 million with proceeds returned to the breast cancer cause nationwide in support of awareness and education, screening and diagnosis, access to treatment, support services, and scientific research.

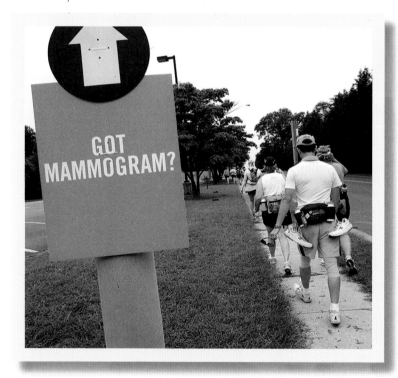

An alternative to the long-distance breast cancer walk is the American Cancer Society's Making Strides Against Breast Cancer series. Approximately 100 Making Strides events now occur around the country each year, usually in or near October, which is National Breast Cancer Awareness Month. Though the designated distance is about five miles, participants are free to walk as long as they can and to take as long as they wish. The events are intended to appeal to people of all ages, and, in some locations, bicyclists, in-line skaters, and even dogs are invited to participate. Unlike the Avon Foundation and Komen Foundation events, there is no preregistration or registration fee. All you've got to do to participate is show up at the event with your completed registration form, whatever money you intend to contribute, and your walking shoes. You'll probably want to bring a few extra dollars to purchase a souvenir T-shirt—a sign of your ongoing support in the fight against breast cancer.

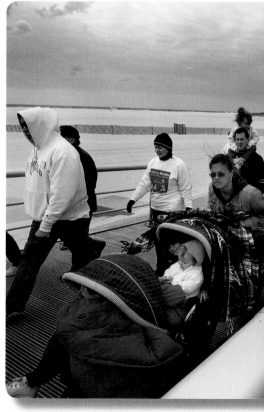

As event organizers like to put it, "There's no minimum required fundraising amount, but there's no maximum either!" The Making Strides series demonstrates, once again, that when it comes to fighting breast cancer, people are mighty generous.

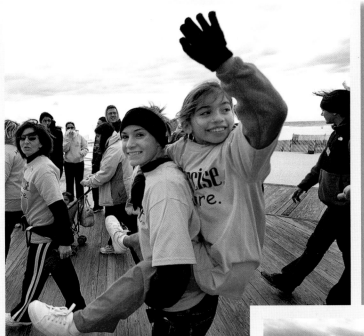

The American Cancer Society is dedicated to eliminating cancer by preventing cancer, saving lives, and diminishing suffering from cancer through research, education, advocacy, and service. At the 2004 Making Strides event on Long Island's Jones Beach, for example, 40,000 walkers turned out on a cold and windy day to raise a total of $2.2 million for the cause.

Over Making Strides' 13-year history, nearly two million walkers across the country have contributed more than $100 million to fight breast cancer on four fronts: to fuel the most promising research, to spread lifesaving breast cancer awareness, to advocate for screening opportunities for all people, and to ease the cancer burden for people facing the disease.

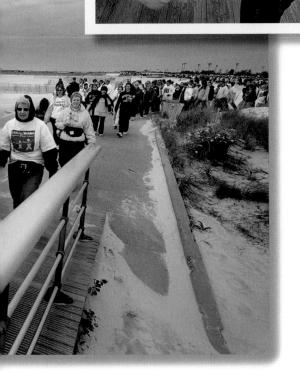

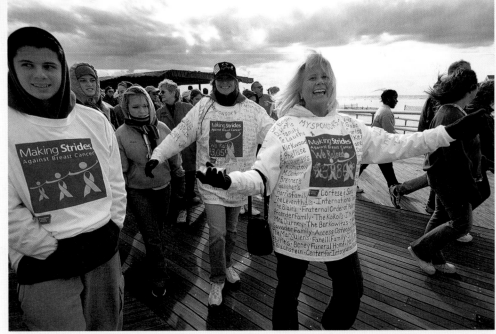

Walking in
Celebration

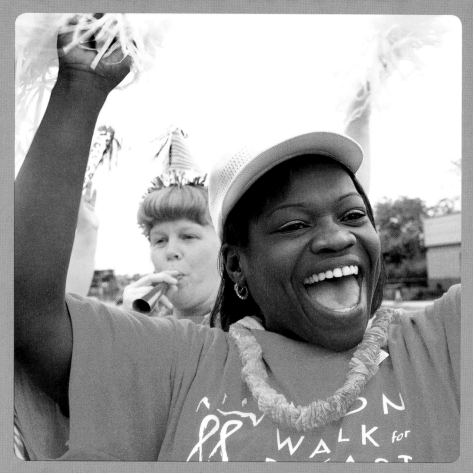

The journey for the person who has been diagnosed with breast cancer is much different from that of the other walkers. The survivors are our true heroes. They know what it means to lose their hair and fight for their lives. Each step they take on this walk is one more step to recovery, and every walker joins in the celebration of another life saved from this dreaded disease. When the rest of us think we just can't go another mile, a walker wearing a "SURVIVOR" shirt inevitably comes into view, and we find the strength to keep on walking. *If they can finish after what they've been through, so can I!*

I walk because...

"Five years after my diagnosis, I still had never taken the time to deal with my cancer emotionally. Walking with my teammates forced me to do that—especially the closing ceremonies, where they honor the survivors. It was incredibly powerful." —*Maria Bradfield*

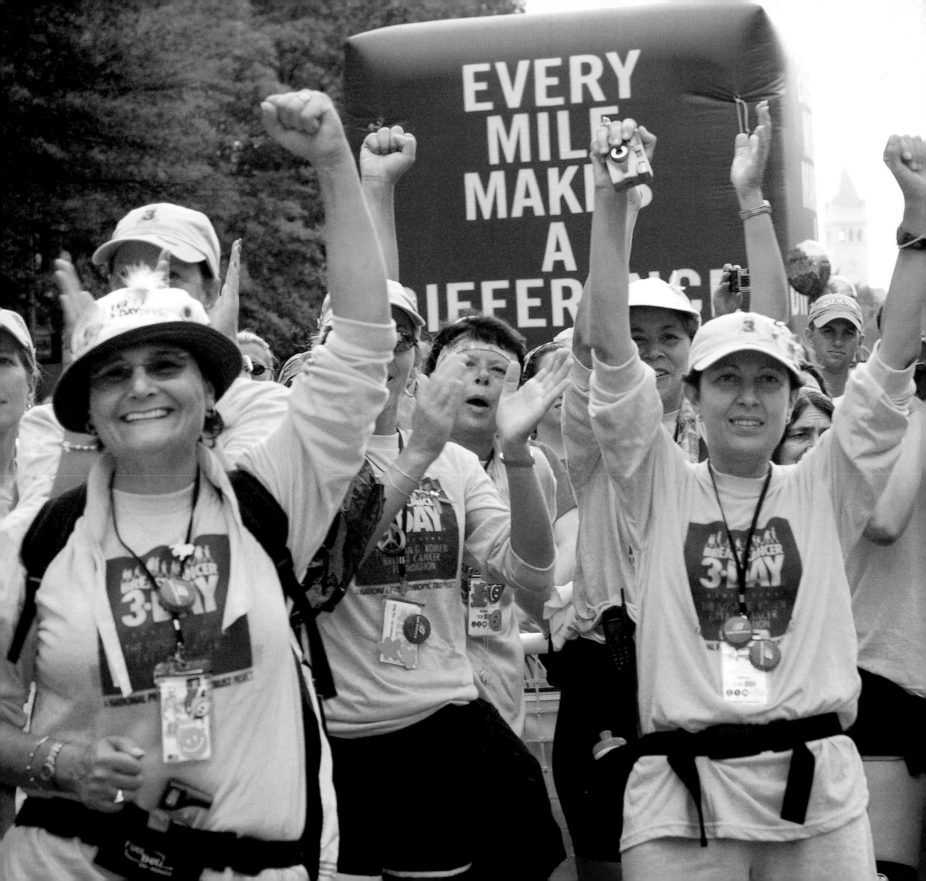

Patty Matthews

Allentown, New Hampshire

"I didn't know what to expect, but Holy cow!—it was incredible."

By all rights, Patty Matthews shouldn't have been participating in the 2004 Avon Walk for Breast Cancer in Boston. She had finished her chemotherapy regimen only a week before the event. As she explains it, "Seven to ten days after a Taxol treatment is the worst time because that's when the side effects start happening." Patty couldn't even feel her feet during the walk, she says, and she was in excruciating pain, but she had a reason for being there that outweighed the agony of her body.

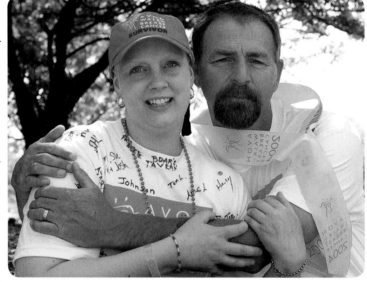

As she tells the story, she was at home during her recovery with her then one-year-old daughter, Mary, and her mother, who was helping take care of the family. Suddenly she realized that a familiar song was playing on the television. It was Vanessa Carlton's "A Thousand Miles," the first song she and her infant daughter heard together when the baby was on the way home from the hospital. "I said at the time that it would always be our song," says Patty. "I actually have the CD in her baby book, along with the lyrics and everything." Mary heard it playing, too, says Patty, and was "kind of dancing" to the music. "Then when I looked at the television, I realized that it was an advertisement for the Avon Walk for Breast Cancer. I never had any idea. I mean, the hair stood up on my arms."

Patty says she had never heard of the Avon Walk for Breast Cancer, but she knew in that instant that she would register and participate. Worried that Patty wouldn't have the strength, her mother asked when the event was to take place. "I said I didn't care when it was. I was going to raise the money, and if I could possibly go, I was going to go. It was a sign. There was a reason that song came on at that moment."

Patty's participation in the walk was an act of courage physically and emotionally. She was only 32 years old when she discovered a lump in her breast. "My doctor

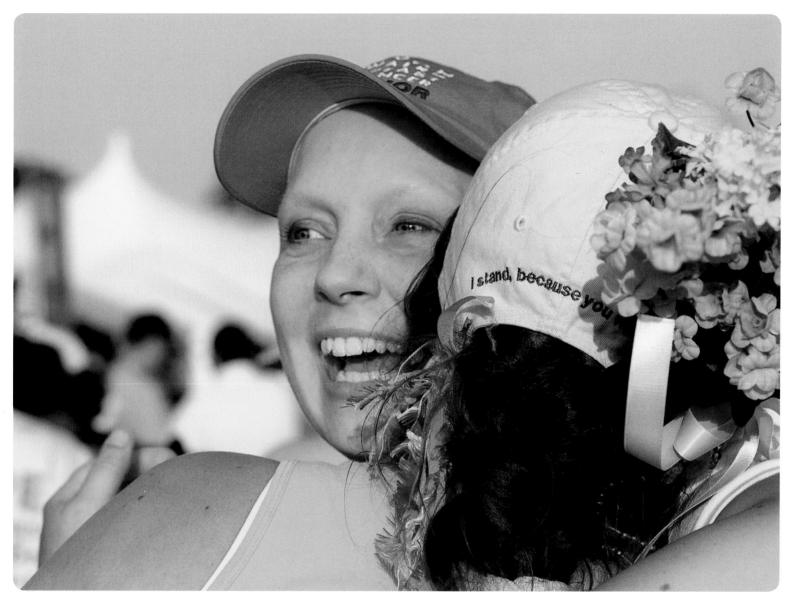

assured me that because I had no family history and because I was so young, there was nothing to worry about. 'We'll do the lumpectomy and everything will be fine,' he said." When she went in for the surgery, says Patty, her physician was still assuring her she had absolutely nothing to worry about. "Well, I woke up after the procedure and saw the doctor moving about a hundred miles an hour past my bed." In fact, she had breast cancer—invasive ductal

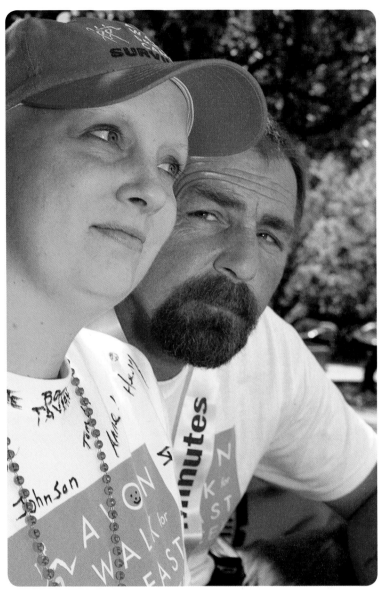

cancer, very aggressive—and she had to be scheduled for a mastectomy as quickly as possible. Patty had her surgery December 26 and started a chemotherapy regimen that lasted until May 7, the week before the Avon Walk.

But Patty says she knows—and knew when she signed up for the walk—that her battle is far from over. In a way, she says, going through the treatment is the easy part. "When you're in treatment you think you're getting well and everything's okay," she says, "but when you have the kind of cancer I have, with a high rate of recurrence, a whole new kind of anxiety sets in. You start thinking, *How long do I have—one year, two years, five years? How long is it going to be before I have to go through that all over again?* And that's reality."

Patty's not the type to shield herself from the truth. She knows that her cancer has an 87 percent chance of recurring, which, as she says, "is not good." As her doctor "so eloquently" put it: "Am I going to see my daughter go to kindergarten? Probably. Am I going to see her graduate from high school? Maybe not."

What happens when you are facing that kind of truth, says Patty, is that "you embrace every minute of every day that you can. Every day to me now is a good day." Then she adds with a laugh, "They're all equally stressful."

Patty describes walking in the Avon Walk as "the most inspirational thing I have ever done—and the hardest." Knowing what the consequences might be if she exhausted herself, she persevered for 10 miles. "I was walking for everybody," she says. "I just saw so many other people who were so much worse than I was—and so many walking in memory of people they had lost—I realized how fortunate I was to be alive. I didn't even think about my own chemo. Being with my friends and my family and seeing everybody else was just awesome."

By the way, those "family and friends" numbered 10 in all, and they all got involved as volunteers. When Patty couldn't walk anymore, she and her entourage proceeded to the T-shirt tent and handed out

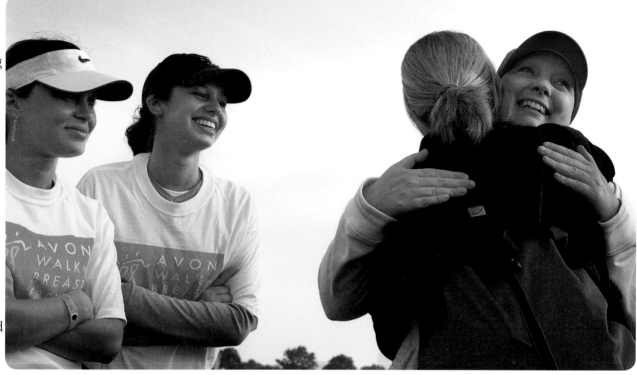

T-shirts to all the walkers. Her mother directed traffic, says Patty, "holding back the crowd and showing everybody where to go for closing ceremonies." Her husband, Chuck, spent the weekend following along to make sure Patty was okay. "But next year," she says, "we're both registered, and we'll walk together."

The reason she'll walk next year "and for the rest of my life," says Patty, "is the positive atmosphere, the incredible energy, and the way it makes you feel." Regardless of whether she was a survivor or not, she would have been amazed at "all the people who put their heart and soul into this—just because it was a good

cause." Patty says she was in tears the whole time, moved by the courage and passion of so many people. "I've never experienced anything like it in my life. I wish I could be exposed to it every day. It was absolutely incredible."

Patty says her only regret is that she didn't become involved earlier. But she understands that it often takes that one person with a personal stake in the battle to get those close to her on board. "That's when you realize it could be you, or your mom, or your sister," says Patty. "The momentum starts building when people realize they don't have to have breast cancer for it to affect them. And pretty soon, something incredible is happening."

Tayra Perez

Burke, Virginia

"It was a matter of getting back to life."

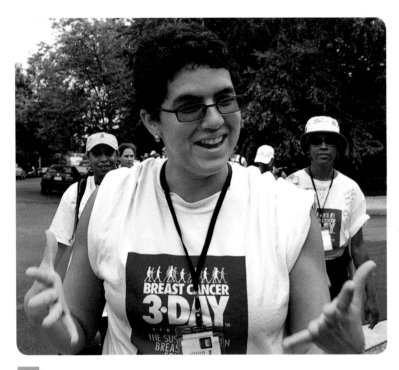

Tayra Perez was breast-feeding her 10-month-old son, Gabriel, when she discovered the lump. "I thought it was just because of the breast-feeding," says Tayra, "but I went and had it checked out and found out I had cancer."

Out of nowhere she found herself in the middle of her worst nightmare—one she says she survived thanks to tremendous family support. Tayra is Puerto Rican; her husband, Robert, is Cuban, and they have "a huge family

on both sides." She credits Robert with "definitely being right there" through it all, helping her keep a positive attitude. But her mother, whom she calls "a pillar of strength," did her husband one better. When Tayra was losing her hair, her mother shaved her own head in solidarity. "It was pretty awesome," says Tayra. "I told her she didn't have to do that. But I went on vacation, and when I got back she picked me up at the airport and she was bald."

By March of 2004, Tayra had finished her chemo and had undergone surgery. Then she saw an announcement for the Breast Cancer 3-Day Walk coming to Washington. She decided to go for it. "I wanted to start a new chapter in my life," she says. "I was cancer-free and wanted to close the book on that part of my life and start a new part with a new challenge. I liked feeling healthy and being able to train. It was a matter of getting back to life."

Not that it was easy. Exercise was never Tayra's thing. But Robert stayed right beside her, not simply encouraging her but training alongside her. "He got up to 20 miles a day with me," she says, and, in fact, he would have loved to walk with her during the event. The only thing that stopped him was that they didn't believe they could raise enough money for both of them to enter.

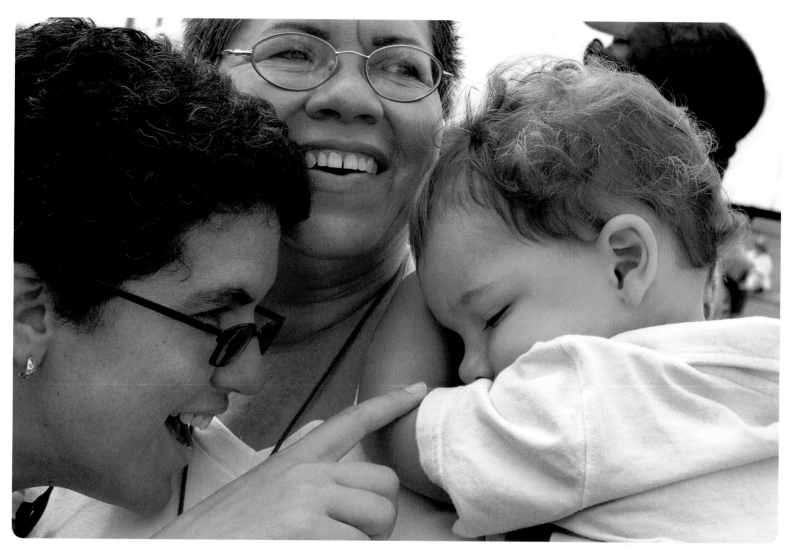

Instead, as happens so often, Tayra found new friends to walk with—including Laura, a 15-year survivor. "There were plenty of times on Day Two that she wanted to quit," says Tayra. "She's like, 'I'm taking the bus.' I'm like, '*No!*' Later, they reversed roles, and Laura was the one who kept Tayra from dropping out. "We encouraged each other

the whole way. We were really proud of walking the whole thing, but we had *so* many blisters."

Actually, Tayra says she was even more impressed by all the people walking who were *not* survivors, the people who were walking for a mother or a sister or loved one. "To see how many people are doing it because they have somebody like me in their family is really amazing," she says, and she also sees how important it is. "You really need that lifeline. You need the support. Even though you think you're strong, you know, after a while your glass just gets full."

The walk also brings another important realization, says Tayra: it puts your own situation into perspective. "You are so shocked at first, so frightened, so aware of your mortality. But then you come out on the other side and you see that what you've been through has been hard, but other people have it so much harder. You're thinking, *I was complaining about this? Look at these people.*"

Ultimately, though, Tayra believes that the Breast Cancer 3-Days are all about raising awareness and raising money. She agrees that there is not enough awareness in the Latin community, but she believes the problem runs deeper than that. "A lot of people are just in denial," she says. "They don't want to know if anything is wrong with them." She cites as an example an uncle of hers who died of prostate cancer. "It wasn't until he was really in pain that he went to the doctor," says Tayra. "Well, it was way too late then."

Other problems, too, make the situation more difficult for Latinos and other minority populations. "Some of the Mexican community are in this country illegally," she notes, "and they think if they go to the hospital they will get in trouble." Many others, who are legal immigrants, simply don't have medical insurance. "My diagnosis was

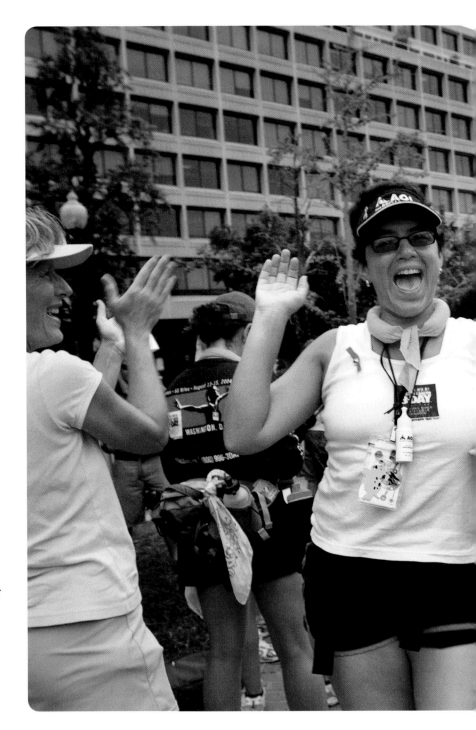

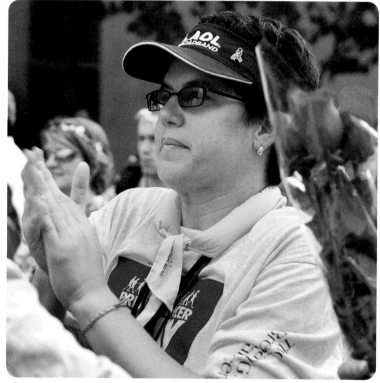

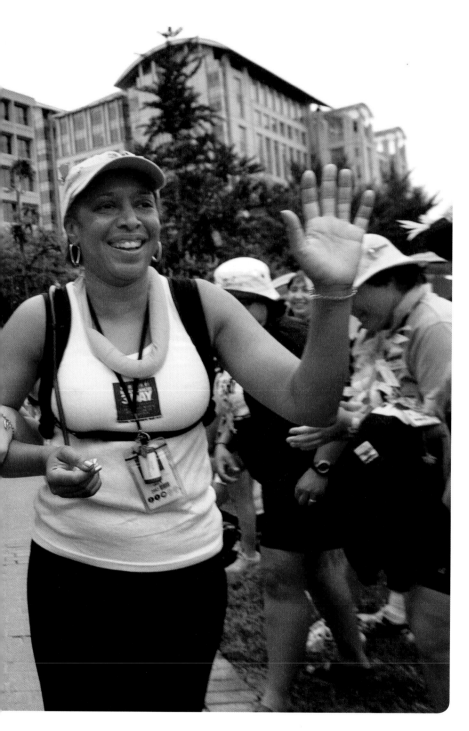

shocking," she says, "but what else is shocking is the bills I see going to my insurance company. I mean, thank God I'm covered, because it's incredible how much it costs."

This, above all, is the reason to walk: "If that money we raised helps just one person, if somebody that doesn't have insurance is able to get a mammogram, that's all that matters."

So is Tayra ready to walk again? "Listen, it was totally worth it. The people I met, and being in that special world for those three days. And it was a great thing for me to finish that long of a distance. But again? Hmmmm . . . maybe a shorter one. I mean, I don't do exercise."

Karen Borkowsky

Program Director, Avon Walk for Breast Cancer

"I get such a high from being up on that stage and looking out at that sea of beautiful people."

Karen Borkowsky's great-grandmother and great-aunt both died of breast cancer. Her mother is a survivor who was diagnosed with the disease in 1987 and underwent a lumpectomy, six months of chemotherapy, and 40 radiation treatments. In 1996, her father's sister discovered she had the disease.

With such a family history, it's not surprising that Karen entered a Memorial Sloan-Kettering breast cancer surveillance program when she turned 30. It seemed a sensible precaution, even though she was in perfect health and her life was wonderful. She had a great career as a shoe buyer for Macy's, she was young and single in fabulous Manhattan, and she was such a "total crazy runner and health freak" that in the summer of 1998 she started training for the New York City Marathon.

In October of that year, right before the marathon, she noticed blood inside her sports bra—no big deal, just chafing or an abrasion, Karen figured. But the doctors at her regular clinical breast exam were concerned about the

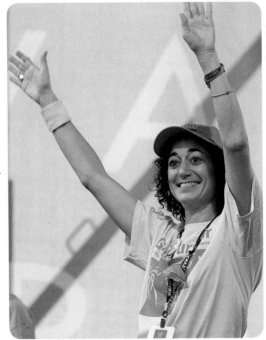

blood. "They told me to go run the marathon and have a good time, but to get a mammogram as soon as it was over." The mammogram found no abnormalities, but a subsequent ductogram and surgery led to the discovery of a tumor.

"It was December 23, 1998," Karen recalls, "when they called to say, 'You have breast cancer.' I was sitting in my office at work, and I think I just started shrieking. Of course, every doctor in Manhattan was off for the holidays, so it was January 4 before I could get an appointment. On January 6, I was on the table for my first mastectomy." A month later she had a second mastectomy, followed by reconstruction and six months of chemotherapy.

If modern medicine saved Karen's life, it's fair to say that Avon saved her mind and spirit. Even with her course of chemotherapy just beginning, she signed up for the 60-mile Avon Breast Cancer 3-Day Walk from Bear Mountain to Central Park, New York, to be held in August 1999. "When I saw the announcement for that 60-mile walk,"

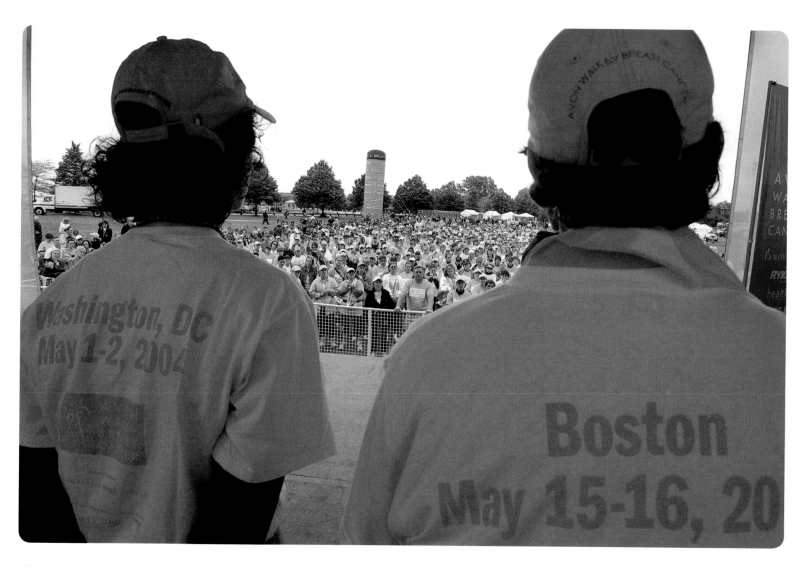

she says, "I knew it was something I had to do. I had been thinking I might never run again, so maybe I needed to prove something to myself."

Karen didn't just train herself for the 60-mile walk. Even though she was sick from the chemo, she volunteered to be a training walk leader, and all through the spring and summer led 8-to-10-mile hikes through Central Park in preparation for the event. She also plunged headlong into fundraising for the event, and instead of the minimum $1,800, she raised $41,000.

In April, a cable TV station interviewed her, then taped her entire training walk, which gave her a chance to share her story for the first time. She found the experience so rewarding that immediately afterward she decided to quit her job. She took a short-term disability leave—enough to get her through the event—but never went back. "I decided I didn't want to be a shoe buyer any more," Karen says with a laugh. "I was meeting all these incredible people. I was getting well. I figured this was what I was supposed to

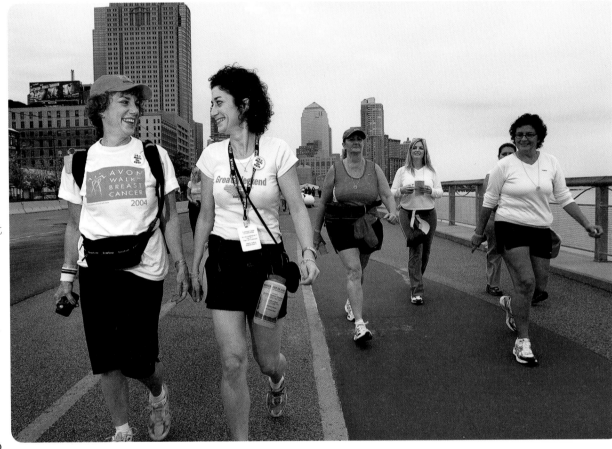

be doing." In October, she interviewed with the American Cancer Society New York and was hired to direct the Society's Making Strides Against Breast Cancer in Central Park, a five-mile fundraising event held every October.

Karen ran the hugely popular Making Strides event for three years before being "called home" to the Avon Foundation at the end of 2003. "Ever since that first 3-Day, I had been interested in working with Avon," Karen explains. "It seemed like the best combination of corporate and non-

profit, and I really admired all the things they were doing for women. I was about to move to California, and I think this was the only job that could have kept me in New York."

The job? Program director for the entire Avon Walk for Breast Cancer series, which in 2004 consisted of six weekend events in cities across the nation. In 2003, the launch year, the Avon Walks raised $25 million, and in 2004 they topped $35 million.

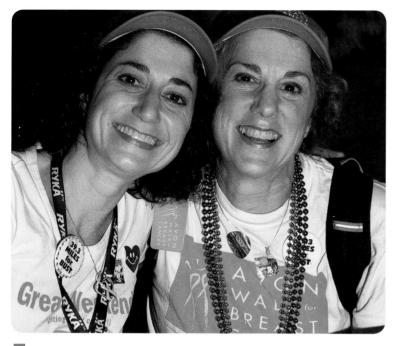

"**T**o me it was so wonderful," says Karen's mother, Judy Borkowsky. "Words fail me because I was just so proud."

Judy had just spent the weekend walking beside her daughter—two cancer survivors together—at the Avon Walk event in New York City. After the first day, 26 miles in a cold rain, Judy says she thought she would never walk again. But after soaking her feet in Epsom salts and getting a good foot massage, she was ready for the second day. "Such a wonderful experience," she says, "even if I did get tired."

For Karen, walking with her mother was the highlight of her five-year involvement in the fight against breast cancer. For Judy, the mother of the event manager, it was even sweeter.

"To see Karen up on that stage and to hear people yelling, 'We love you, Karen'—well, that was pretty amazing."

But it wasn't the end of the story.

A couple of days after the event, an e-mail arrived at Avonwalk.org with the subject line, "This is for Karen Borkowsky." The e-mail read: *I think I had your mother as a fourth-grade teacher in Commack, Long Island, in 1964. I saw you [Karen] on television last night on Channel 4 news, and you look just like her, and the name is not that familiar. If she is that woman, will you please tell your mom that she was a wonderful teacher and I have very fond memories of my fourth-grade class.* The note was signed "Karen Phillips."

It turns out that Judy remembered little Karen very well. "She was a darling little girl—lovely and charming and smart and just a natural leader." Judy also remembered that she was pregnant with her first child at the time, and that she and her husband were right in the middle of the name-selection process. If the baby turned out to be a girl, Judy decided that she could do no better than name her for "the darling little girl" in her class. "And this is the very person who e-mails Karen 40 years later. Isn't that just unbelievable?"

Somehow it's not surprising that Karen's mother would be the kind of teacher whose students would remember her 40 years later. Great teachers make a difference. Judy's daughter obviously has the same high aspiration.

Jeff Elmore

Norfolk, Virginia

"My message to other men is to get out there and get involved. Stop trying to hide or protect yourself from something you know exists."

Jeff Elmore became a training walk leader because he didn't want anybody else to have the kind of experience he'd had. When he signed up for his first breast cancer event four years ago, he'd blown off the training. He hadn't known anybody in the Norfolk area to train with, and Washington was three and a half hours away. "It was hard to get motivated to drive that far for the training walks," he recalls. "Besides, my attitude was, *I can do this—no big deal*."

Jeff says he ended up hurting himself so badly he was in pain for two weeks afterward. "I had to go to the doctor to have X-rays to make sure I didn't have shin splints."

Worse than the pain, though, was his realization that he had really missed out on the essence of the experience. "I was in so much pain that I couldn't focus on what the whole thing was about—the camaraderie and the great messages the walkers were trying to get across." When it was over, he says, he went into his tent to nurse his aching bones and didn't come out, didn't socialize with anybody. He began to realize what he had missed when he started reading all the e-mails and Internet postings about what a great event it had been.

After it was over, his first thought had been, *I'm never doing that again*. But when the time came to sign up for the next year's event, his thinking changed to, *I'm never doing it* wrong *again*. He gathered other interested Norfolk people together and took on the job of training leader. He had realized what the event should be—and what it should not be. "I wanted everybody to get everything out of it—to have the feeling that it would all be okay, to be confident that they could enjoy it."

As for his own experience that second year, Jeff says it was like night and day. "It was so much better. I could focus on the event, on the people, the spirit of the thing. I never had a blister, never had a bit of pain, just because I was so much better prepared that time around." It was also gratifying, he says, when none of his people "had to come in on a wheelchair or a stretcher."

Jeff walks in honor of his mother, who was diagnosed 15 years ago, when Jeff was 14. "I had no clue at the time," he says. "She sheltered us from it completely. I don't think I could have dealt with it. Basically you had a very young, healthy woman who was absolutely incapacitated for several weeks. She had a double mastectomy."

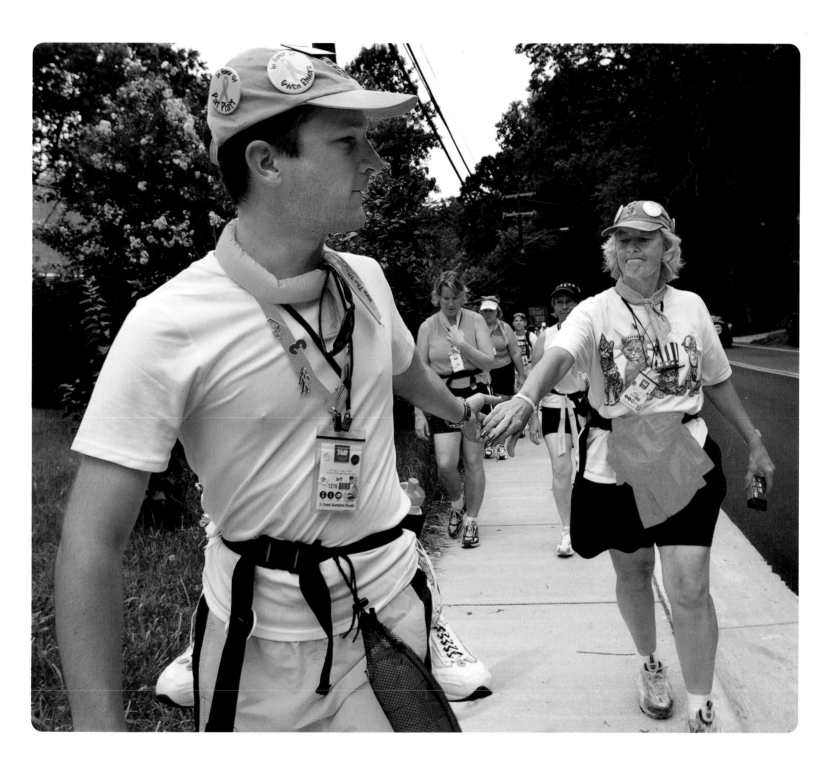

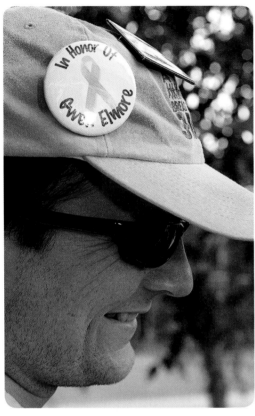

He still admires the strength she showed at the time, and his participation in the fight against breast cancer has brought them closer. She is proud of him, of course, and always comes to the closing ceremonies. But perhaps more important, they can now talk about what she went through. "Her whole concern at the time," says Jeff, "was not what would happen to her but what would happen to her children. Now it scares me, it just really scares me to think that she might not have been here."

Getting in touch with emotions like those is very much a part of what these events are all about, Jeff believes—especially for men. "It's very refreshing," he says. "In everyday life men are supposed to be strong and not cry, not have emotions, but at any of these events you can cry and nobody cares. You can be who you are."

He remembers that second year, when he had trained hard and made it through the event pain-free. "I got to the end and everything was hunky-dory. I was just sitting there eating my lunch, happy as could be, and all of a sudden it was like somebody opened the floodgates.

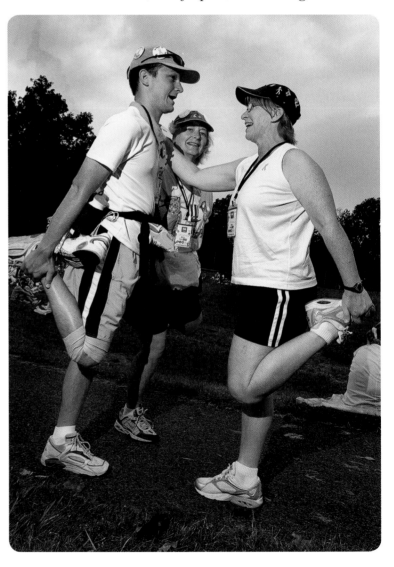

Nothing really triggered it that I recall. Maybe I found myself looking at a survivor or something. But all of a sudden I realized that what we were doing really did make a difference, and, man, that was it for me."

Call it empathy—the ability to share, deeply, what other people are going through. Jeff says that in this year's event he found himself hurting on Day Two because on Day One he wore the wrong shoes. "My feet were killing me. But then I started talking to a woman who had just been diagnosed, and as I listened to her story, all of a sudden my feet weren't hurting anymore. That made the walk so much more meaningful for me, because she was so alive and so determined that it wasn't going to beat her."

Jeff will agree, though, that it does take a certain kind of man to participate—one who is comfortable with his sexuality, one who can speak frankly with women, one with a broad mind. And most important, says Jeff with a laugh, "You can't be afraid to wear pink."

He would love to see more men out there. After all, if enough guys showed up, he points out, they would have to provide more than one shower stall for men. More seriously, Jeff has a message to the men who are hanging back: "Get involved," he says. "Stop trying to hide or protect yourself from something that you know exists."

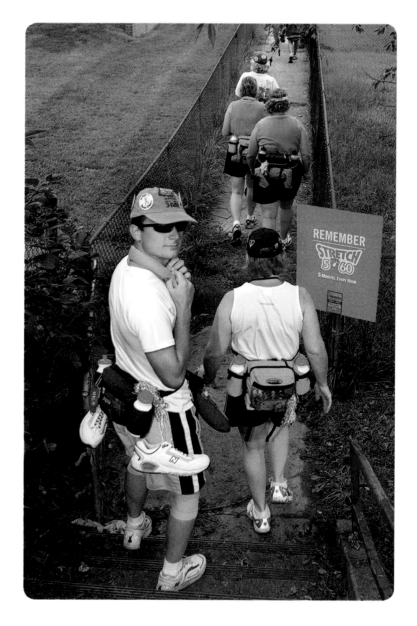

Kimber Peterson & Nancy Jennings

San Francisco, California

"It's just really nice to know that you're not alone after all, and Kimber and I basically feel like we're going through this together." —*Nancy Jennings*

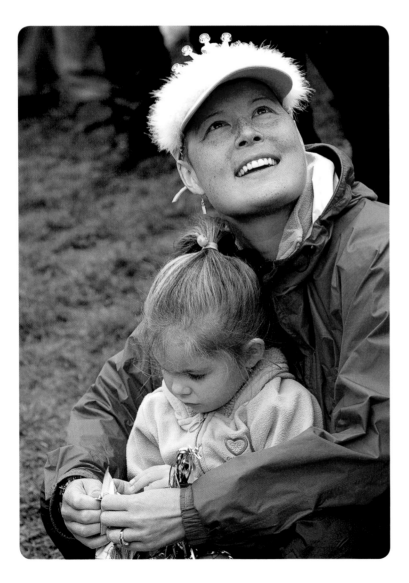

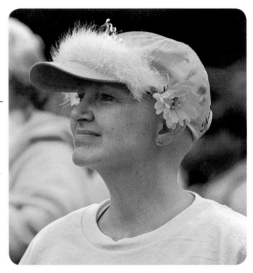

For 10 years Nancy Jennings had talked about getting breast reduction surgery. When she finally got HMO approval, she underwent the procedure in December 2003. "I was so excited about having a different body," says 40-year-old Nancy. "It was going to be the year of the pretty boobs."

But during the follow-up, the serious expression on the face of her plastic surgeon—"normally a very bubbly guy"—told Nancy all was not well. The routine biopsy of the tissue taken from her body revealed breast cancer. "All of a sudden he's talking about a mastectomy," Nancy recalls, "and I just lost it." Worse yet, the completed pathology report indicated cancer in both breasts. "So I go from thinking I'm going to have pretty boobs to talking about a double mastectomy in a matter of days."

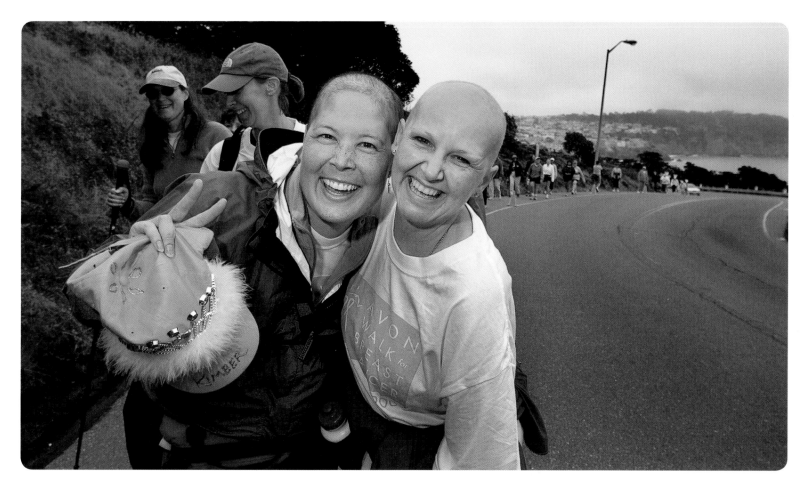

A month later, in January 2004, an equally devastating surprise awaited Kimber Peterson. Out of the blue, the 37-year-old wife and mother of two was diagnosed with stage 3B breast cancer. "It's pretty aggressive," says Kimber. "But it's like when I'm doing extreme skiing and standing on terrain that scares me. I just look into it, take a breath, and jump in . . . ski hard and don't miss any turns. I'm doing the same with my cancer treatment."

Unknown to each other at the time they were diagnosed, the two women are now closer than sisters, thanks to a mutual friend who was gathering a group of women to participate in the Avon Walk for Breast Cancer in San Francisco. Nancy signed up first, then tried to talk Kimber into joining the team. "She said she had already thought about doing it, but her doctors had told her '*no!*' She was scheduled to finish her chemo right before the walk." Then, a few days later, says Nancy, she got an e-mail back from Kimber saying, "Screw it. I'm doing it!"

Kimber says that the mutual friend, Kristen, was the ringleader and the one who first encouraged her. "But Nancy pushed me over the edge." It was Nancy who pointed out that they had buses running, that if Kimber was too weak to make it, she didn't have to. "I thought, well, if I don't have to do the whole thing, I'll go for it."

The two women formed an uncommon bond. As Nancy puts it, "When you first get your diagnosis, you feel so alone, it's like you're speaking this language that no one else can understand. It's just really nice to know that you're not alone after all, and Kimber and I basically feel like we're going through this together."

As for the Avon Walk itself, both found the experience unforgettable—and healing in ways they couldn't have foreseen. "I was so focused on myself," says Nancy. "All I could think about was how I was feeling, my next appointment, all the paperwork. The walk brings you out of that tunnel and gives you a sense of the greater community. You're in touch with other people." In fact, Nancy says she was so depressed toward the end of her chemo that her friends worried about how withdrawn she had become. "The five weeks we spent training and then doing the walk just brought me back to life." Kimber adds that the experience of the walk helps you to see the experience of the disease itself in a whole new perspective. "You're able to put your whole life in a new context," she says. "I'm closer to my husband now. I enjoy my kids more, my job. I face life now going, *Oh, cool, it's another day*." In other words, the walk

allows you to achieve "a kind of peace you would have never found if you hadn't gone through this experience."

Nancy and Kimber also agree that the Avon Foundation does an effective job of making the threat of breast cancer—and the fight against it—"very real and tangible." Kimber was especially impressed by the idea of putting a pink ribbon on a different walker every three minutes—i.e., the same interval at which a new case of breast cancer is diagnosed. "First you see a few ribbons," says Kimber. "Then you start to see a lot of ribbons, and by the end of the event you see a sea of ribbons. That really hits home—a great testimony about how cancer spreads through a population." Nancy was particularly moved by the fact that much of the money raised by the event is distributed right then—during closing ceremonies. "To see specifically where the money was going, and to see that it was being used locally, I thought that was really wonderful."

The sense of fun, of joy, and of celebration that Kimber and Nancy exhibited throughout the event was evident to anyone walking in their proximity. Part of it, says Nancy, is that both women just happened to have a great sense of humor. "Another part is that we like to make fun of our cancer as a way to get back at it, a way to control it." There's plenty that you can't control, she says, but one thing you can control is your attitude. "Just comparing stories about how lousy your taste buds have gotten, or how horrible your hair looks—it's a huge help to be able to laugh at these things."

But both of these courageous women know that the

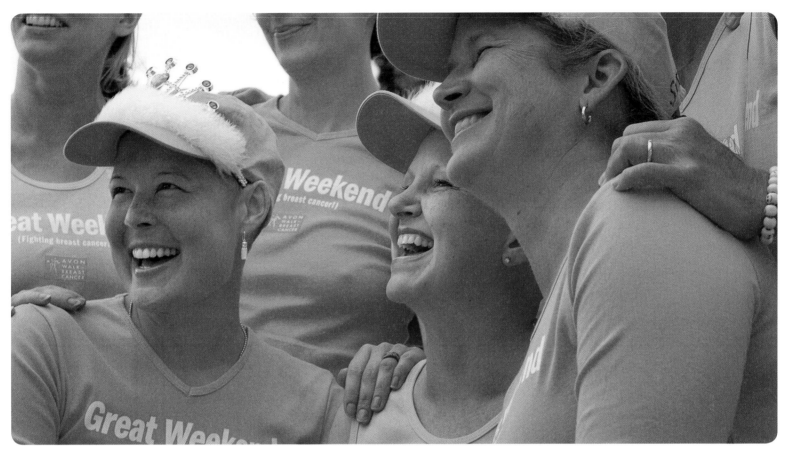

battle is far from over—not for breast cancer victims generally, nor for themselves in particular. Kimber is facing another round of chemo and is only half through with her radiation treatments. "The doctors can't really tell you if you are cured or not," she says. "There is no test that will say, 'You have no cancer.' This terribly uncertain situation is made even more complicated when you have a small daughter who wonders why your hair is falling out, but, as Kimber puts it, "in my case, we are working with the assumption that it's gonna work out."

As for Nancy, she says she is a bit disconcerted when people refer to her as a survivor. She says she's not one of those people who, if they make it to the five-year mark, will have probably beaten the disease. Her type of breast cancer is "slow-growing," she says, and could just as easily recur 20 or 30 years down the road.

"So I really don't know the right word for myself," says Nancy. "But hey, I'm going to fight it. I'm going to be positive and optimistic. Then, when I'm 80, I'll call myself a survivor."

Tim Day
Washington, D.C.

"I'm going to continue until I don't have to anymore."

When Tim Day was a 17-year-old high school student, he noticed a painful lump in his breast. He mentioned it to the doctor at his annual pre-sports physical but got no response. Six months later, when it had grown to be visibly noticeable and so painful that it hurt to have a T-shirt over it, he was still getting no response. So he changed doctors. The new physician biopsied the lump, saw the results, and immediately scheduled surgery.

"He told me I had breast cancer, and I literally went from the doctor's office to the operating room," recalls Tim. "I woke up without really understanding what had happened. All I remember was having the worst pain of my life."

It was far from over. Next came the sickness and nausea that accompany chemotherapy and radiation. Then, exactly a year after he had completed his treatment, the cancer recurred in his other breast. "My only thought was that I could not go through it again." But he did. He had to. Tim had had a second radical mastectomy before he was 20 years old.

Now it was up to him to deal with the scars . . . and the silence.

Growing up in a household with a single mom and three siblings, Tim wasn't encouraged to lean on the family for support. He wasn't encouraged to talk about what he was going through. Not that it would have been easy, under the best of circumstances, for a boy to talk about having breast cancer. "We never discussed it," he says. "Never discussed it with family, never discussed it with friends. Never discussed it at all."

The recurrence was even worse. "More aggressive," says Tim. "Longer chemo and longer radiation. I was extremely sick." But he still got no support. "The family's attitude was that this was my problem and they didn't need to hear about it. So they didn't. I muddled through."

The scarring added another dimension to Tim's isolation. He went for years without ever taking off his shirt in front of another person. "I could be six-two, weigh 190, without an ounce of body fat," he says, "and I still wouldn't take off my shirt. Who would, with a scar under both breasts from armpit to sternum?"

The walls began to come down in 1998. By that time he had become a medical professional, working as a physician's assistant in an oncology practice. One of his patients wanted very badly to participate in an upcoming Avon Breast Cancer 3-Day. The problem was, she was dying. "'What are we going to do?' she asked me. I told her that I

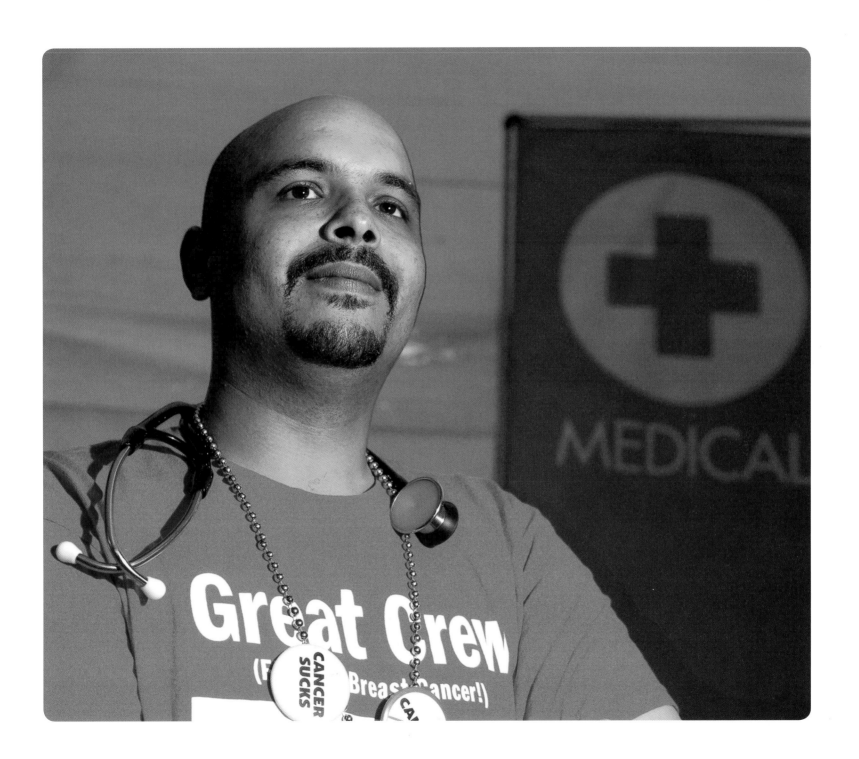

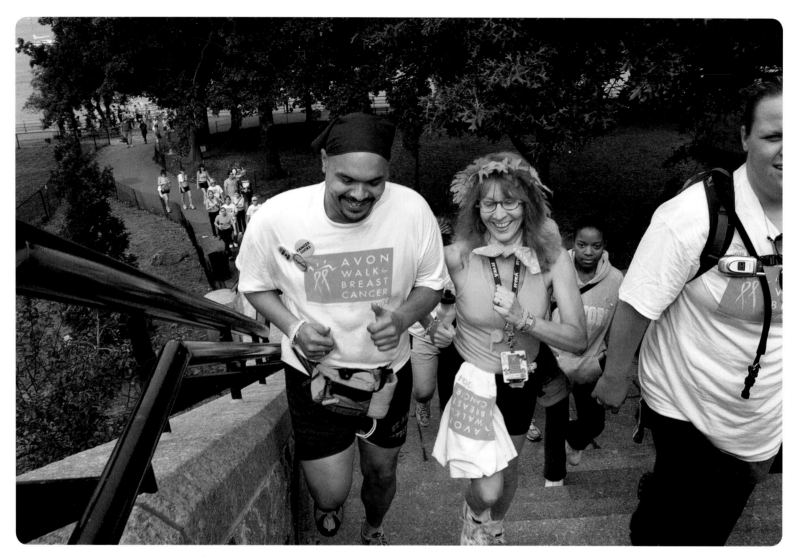

would walk it for her." There wasn't much time left, but between the two of them, they raised "a ton of money," and Tim entered the event.

Although he remembers that first cancer walk as "the most moving experience of my life," Tim still wasn't ready. "It's funny," he says. "There is so much sharing and so much learning going on. Everybody has a story. You learn that the disease affects everyone—young, old, white, black, Asian, wealthy, poor. Everyone has an experience to share. As for me, the first woman I talked to teased me about being there just to 'meet women.' And the only thing I had to share was, 'No, for a lot of reasons, I'm not here to meet women.' Basically, I was still doing my best to stay away from people."

After that walk, though, Tim gradually came to the realization that if he really wanted to help the patients in his office, he needed to help himself first. "You need to be happy with yourself first of all," he says. "I realized I needed to come out about my own cancer. I needed to deal with it. I needed to understand it. I was a grown man working in a field I didn't even understand myself."

It was another three years before Tim made his peace with the disease, and again it was thanks to participation in an Avon Breast Cancer 3-Day. "It was in the last walk of 2001, I believe, and I remember thinking, *I'm going to do this again*. And I did. I signed up on the last day to do the next year's event."

The reason? Tim had finally allowed the environment of the walk to work its magic upon him. He finally felt at ease. "I just knew that I was in a really comfortable place," he says. "I could take a shower without anybody going 'Oh, what's that?' I could say, feel, cry, do whatever I wanted to do. I could let out all the emotions that were inside me wherever I was—whether walking or crewing or just sitting in a tent." Nobody was going to tell him not to discuss it. He had been touched, and in a way he couldn't before, he could touch others.

Now Tim is in the vanguard of the crusade. He has participated in 28 Avon breast cancer walks, whether as a walker, a crew member, or—as is more often the case

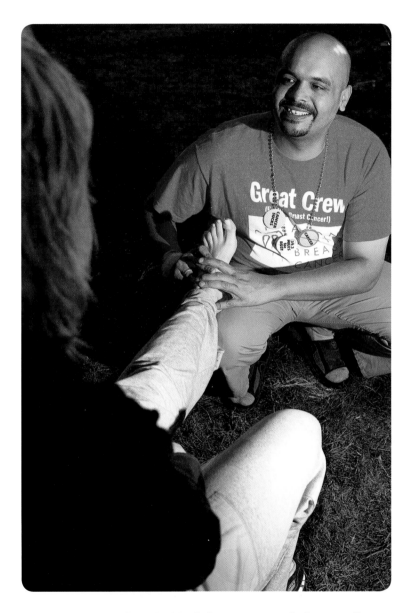

these days—working behind the scenes to help coordinate the medical support.

"And I'm going to continue," says Tim, "until I don't have to anymore."

Monica & Dale Cooper

Oak Hill, Virginia

"This is not just your mother's disease." —*Monica Cooper*

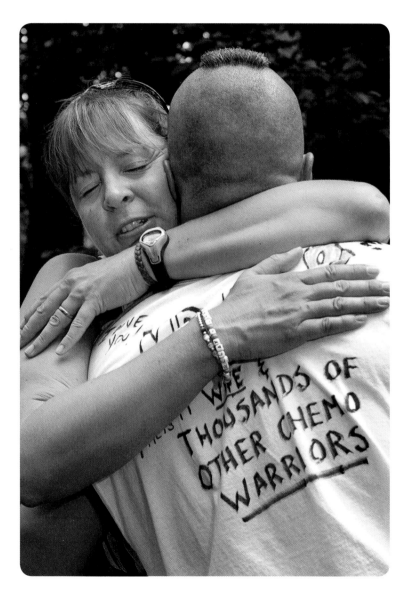

Why do thousands walk together in the fight against breast cancer? Of the countless reasons, one is particularly simple: some things you shouldn't have to go through alone. That's why Monica Cooper first walked in the Komen Race for the Cure®; her best friend had lost her mother to breast cancer, and Monica wanted to be there for her, to share her loss, to help her through her grief.

Her own family was untouched by the disease, and she herself was too young to be threatened by it. So when Monica noticed a pronounced lump in her breast in the fall of 2000, she just "blew it off." After all, she had just started a new job in September. She was too busy to be thinking about health issues. She also blew off her regularly scheduled mammogram in October. "I'm too young for this," Monica told herself. "It has to be nothing. I'm healthy as a horse." She was not only in great shape; she was such a devoted athlete that she had just started kickboxing. And there was no history of cancer in her family. In other words, says Monica, "I was in complete denial."

In February, her husband Dale insisted that she go for her mammogram. "I took my mom with me," Monica recalls, "because as soon as I made the appointment I was thinking to myself, *This is not going to be good*." It wasn't.

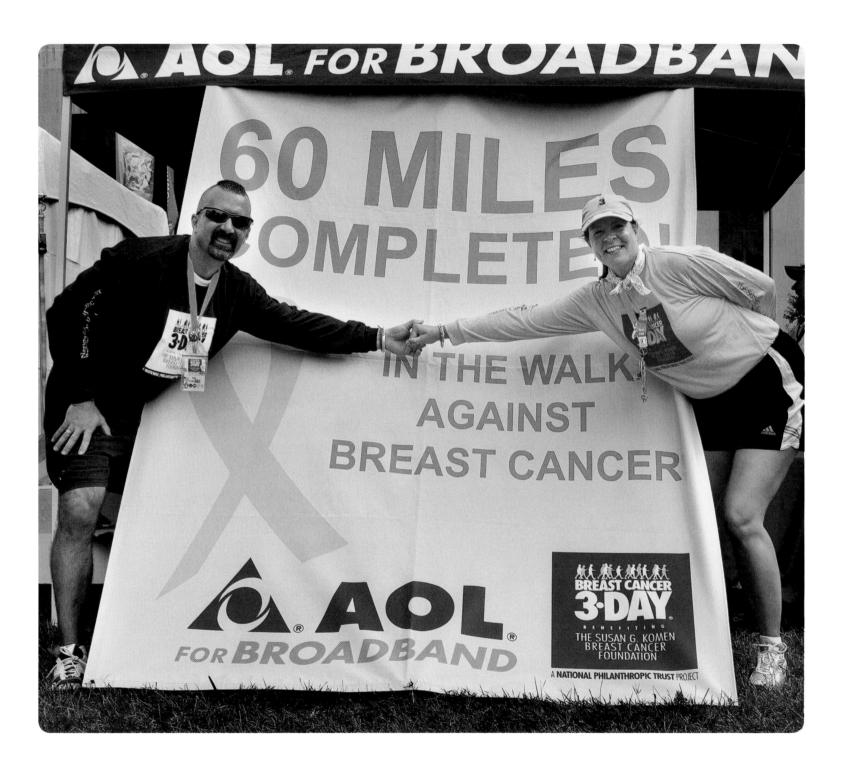

When the procedure was over, the doctor advised her to see an oncologist immediately. "She said it wasn't up to her to make a diagnosis, but she was 95 percent sure I had breast cancer."

On February 9, 2001, a biopsy confirmed her cancer, and she immediately started chemo to shrink her tumors and stop the spread of the disease. On the day before the Komen Race for the Cure®—which she would have to miss for the first time in 10 years—she had a mastectomy. "My best friend had to walk for me that day," she says. Chemo and radiation followed the surgery, with her last chemo treatment, ironically, on September 11, 2001. Her drug regimen was working so well that she started training for

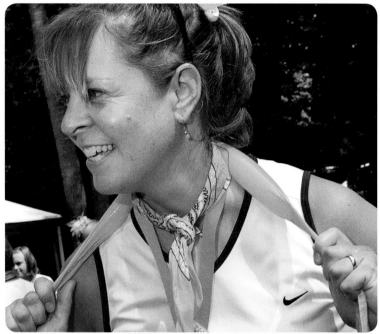

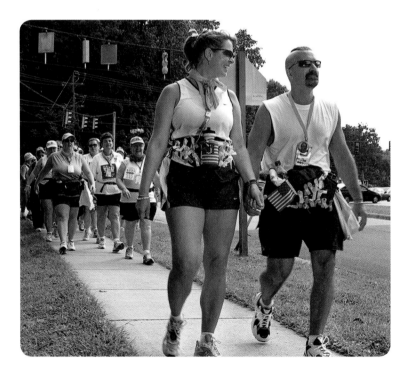

the Breast Cancer Triathlon. "I bought a great bike and was training with my son," says Monica, but then she fell off her bike and injured her shoulder.

She didn't know how bad the injury was, but when it wasn't any better after a couple of days, she went to see an orthopedic surgeon. He told her, sure enough, the shoulder was broken. He also said that Monica had "a lot of other stuff going on in there, but it's probably just swelling." That summer, with the shoulder presumably healed, she was going down a water slide with her kids and heard a big pop in her upper arm. "It was all I could do to get out of the pool," she says, "and then I passed out from the pain." She had broken another bone in her shoulder. When she told her oncologist about it, the doctor immediately ordered a CAT scan. The results: metastasis. She now had cancer in her shoulder and in her ribs. "That started Round Two," says Monica.

It's been difficult for Monica and her family. "At our age," says Dale, a computer consultant, "we're not supposed to be dealing with this. We're supposed to be on vacation, having fun, no cares in the world. And all of a sudden this gets thrown in our lap and changes everything. You're like, 'It's not supposed to be this way,' but it is this way, and now we're faced with it. It has not been fun, and it is not easy."

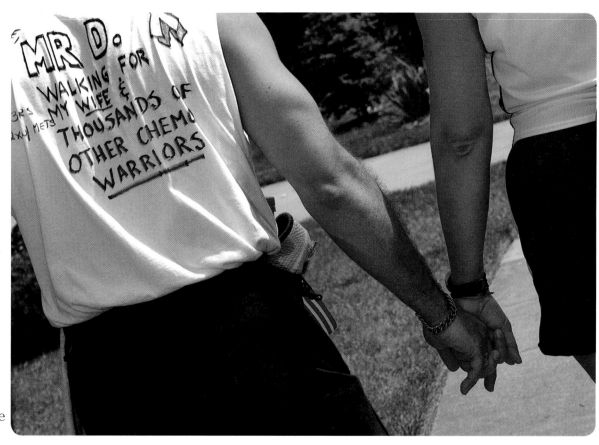

They are both aware of the strain that the disease puts on a marriage. The diagnosis changes your life completely, says Monica, "even your relationship with your husband and children." She points out that even when the victim survives, her marriage usually doesn't: "Something like 60 percent end in divorce."

That's one of the reasons, Monica says, that they decided to walk together in the Breast Cancer 3-Day in Washington, D.C., in August 2004. She had walked the Avon Breast Cancer 3-Day after she was first diagnosed and had crewed the following year, but, she says, "I had always walked with my girlfriend. Dale was always watching the kids."

"That was my job at the time," says Dale. "I needed to focus on keeping the family intact and keeping the kids focused on what they needed to focus on."

"But after my cancer came back," says Monica, "we decided that this walk is for us—to show our commitment to fighting this together."

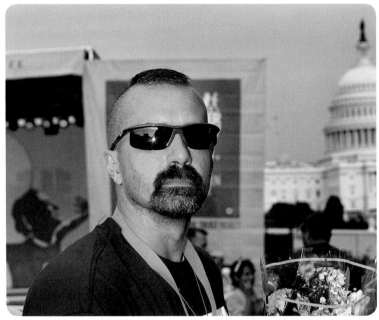

with Monica," he says, "and also an expression of warrior spirit. This was something we had to fight together."

Which is exactly the point of the walk. No one has to fight alone. It's a community of souls, of soldiers, a community breathing a spirit so indomitable that each person's own pain is at least temporarily subsumed in something larger. "I was walking with this woman," says Monica. "She was bald and had just had a double mastectomy, and she said, 'Can I give you a hug—just to thank you for walking for me?' That's exactly why I walk. I'm not walking for me. I'm walking for other people. Every ache and pain you have is nothing when you hear someone else's story. That's why you do it."

For Dale, walking the Breast Cancer 3-Day with Monica signaled the end of his own denial. "It was incredible," he says. "A real turning point. I had been running and running away from this for the past three and a half years, and it was time to step up to the plate. Not getting really involved in the battle had been a big failing on my part."

Monica had lost her hair during her treatment, so for the Breast Cancer 3-Day Walk, Dale cut his off, too—except for a short, Mohawk-like strip along the top. "It was solidarity

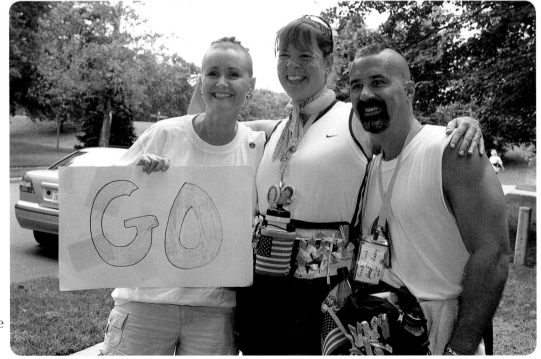

Unfortunately, Monica's own battle wasn't over. Shortly after the Breast Cancer 3-Day in August, a CAT scan revealed some cancer in her lower back. "I told the doctor I felt like I was living from scan to scan," says Monica, "waiting for the bomb to drop. She agreed that, basically, that's what I'm doing. Statistically, I have a 20 percent chance of doing well. Usually it comes back—I guess more aggressively."

Dale adds that Vioxx was the only medication that gave Monica any relief. "Of course, they yanked it off the market. So we're back to square one. She's enduring more pain than anybody should have to go through in life."

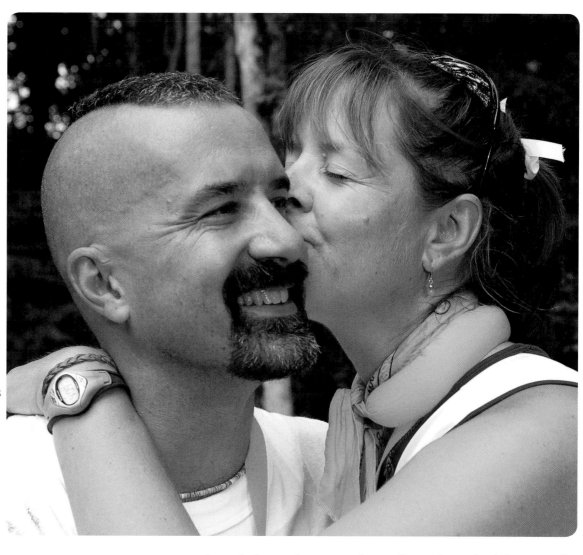

"Yeah," Monica agrees, "it really has been three years of hell. You know, this is not just your mother's disease."

But even still, incredibly, Monica's focus is not on her own pain. She says that her battle with cancer has provided her with "a burden and a gift. You have a knowledge and an experience that others don't have, and you can share that."

Now Monica's only wish is that she were doing more. "I have time now," she says. "I should be outreaching more."

This is the spirit behind the battle against breast cancer. This is why they walk.

Hope

It isn't hard to spot a survivor in the group. They're likely to be wearing a pink baseball hat or T-shirt with "SURVIVOR" imprinted on it. Why do they wear that clothing so proudly? Because they've beaten it! Some have just finished chemo; others might be 20-year survivors. Some accept the personal challenge to be able to say, "I'm back—look what I've done!" Others walk in the hope that none of their loved ones will ever have to hear the words "You have cancer." In every case, they are our inspiration.

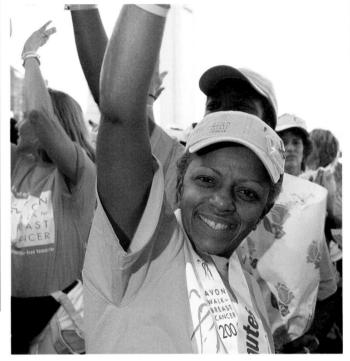

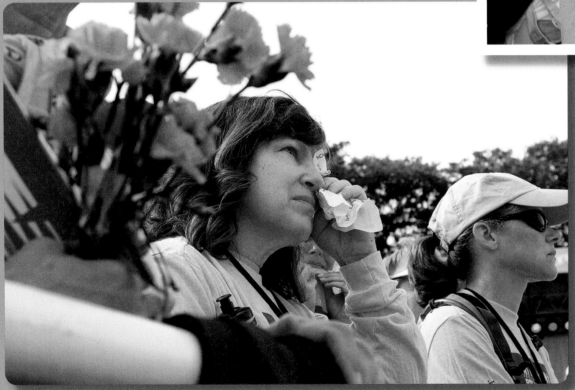

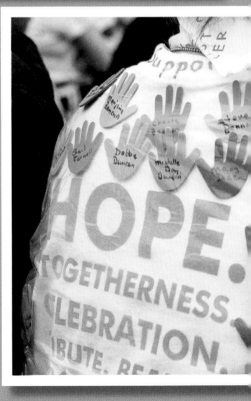

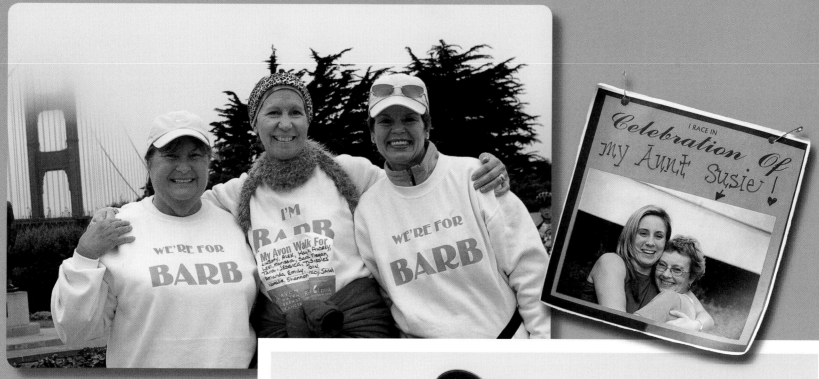

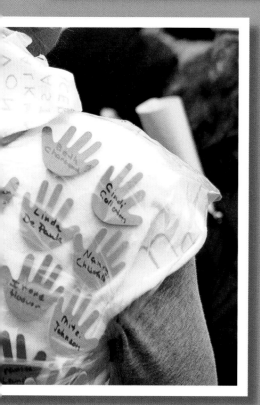

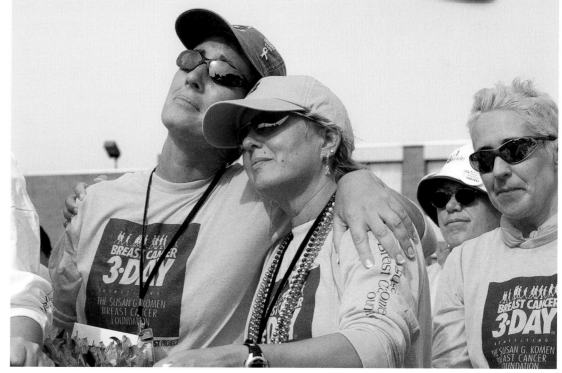

Jennifer Lee

Tecumseh, Michigan

"I get very angry when I hear people say, 'Oh, you are too young to have had breast cancer.'"

Jennifer Lee says people ask her why she has to walk 60 miles. What's wrong with just 5 miles, they ask, or maybe 10 at most? "I tell them it's because it's all about the experience. It's about the suffering, it's about going through something hard for a long time. The pain you are enduring on that walk is very similar to the pain your heart felt during your treatment. And you are going to survive those 60 miles just like you are going to survive breast cancer."

Jennifer speaks from experience. She had a cyst removed from her left breast as a young woman, and because the resulting scar tissue made a routine breast examination more difficult, her doctor suggested a "baseline mammogram" when Jennifer was 26 years old. The test revealed "a circular darkened area" in her right breast, but her doctor was "pretty confident" it was a cyst—"nothing to worry about." She had it checked every three months "to make sure it hadn't changed." After the third checkup, it still hadn't changed, and at that point her doctor's report read, "Follow up with mammogram at age 40 unless other concerns develop."

Two years later, Jennifer returned to the doctor because she felt a nagging, dull ache in that same breast. This time her mammogram lasted three hours, says

Jennifer, because "they took picture after picture after picture." Then she had an ultrasound, after which the radiologist came in. "Normally you don't see them, so that was a little unusual." The radiologist explained that Jennifer had "quite a few areas of calcification" that weren't there two years earlier, along with "a mass in the back." Jennifer says she looked on the screen and saw the same dark spot "that two years ago they said was nothing, but now it was a big spot and they were saying it was something."

Jennifer still assumed it was a cyst, but the radiologist had a different opinion. "What she said was, 'I'm pretty sure you have early breast cancer,'" recalls Jennifer. The mass was biopsied, and a few days later the surgeon confirmed the diagnosis: "We have a small cancer here. Can you come in tomorrow?"

At this point, says Jennifer, her breast cancer education began. "I still wasn't all that concerned," she says. "I thought the surgery would take care of it. I thought they would just fix it—cut it out or kill it with drugs. I really didn't know how deadly breast cancer could be." She was alarmed to hear the surgeon recommend a mastectomy "because there were little spots of cancer all around and he wanted to make sure he got it all." But she

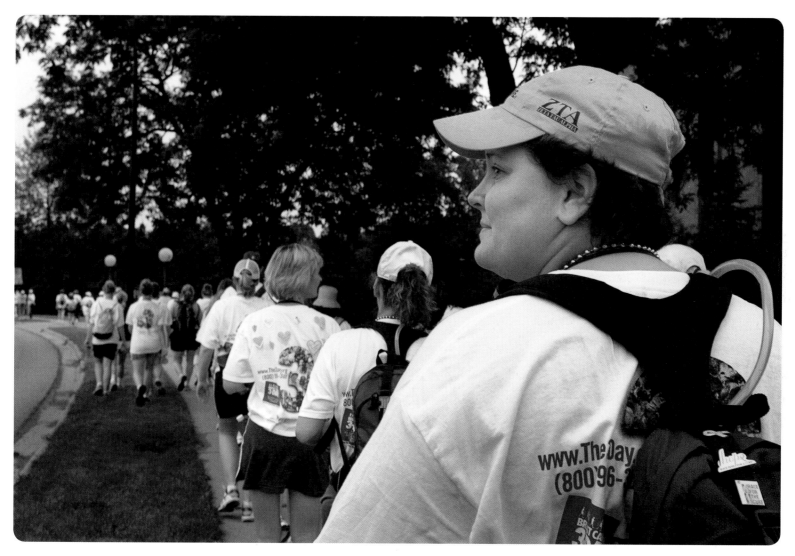

agreed to the plan and had her surgery in May 2003. "I came out of it feeling pretty good," she says. "Not physically but mentally—just because I was thinking the whole thing was over."

When the full pathology report was complete, however, Jennifer says the surgeon came in "with a terrified look on his face." He told her they had removed 18 lymph nodes, 14 of which were full of cancer. "One of them was so enlarged, it was bigger than the original big tumor itself."

That's when Jennifer hit bottom. "I can't describe that feeling," she says. "It's like when you're so heartbroken you can actually feel your heart ache—really, really feel it.

That's what it was like." Jennifer says that when she met with the oncologist, she literally begged him, "Just promise you can give me 20 years so I can raise my children. That's all I want." Of course, the oncologist could make no such promise. "He can only do what he can do," says Jennifer. "That was pretty hard."

Jennifer considers herself "blessed" to have made it through chemo and radiation without the really severe side effects that many people experience. Still, when she heard a woman on the radio talking about a 60-mile breast cancer walk, she was stunned. "I was just at the end of my treatment," she says, "and I was thinking, *No way*." But at the same time, the idea had tremendous appeal. "The woman was saying she was walking for a friend who had breast cancer, and that compared to what her friend was going through, walking 60 miles was nothing. It was awesome." She participated in the Komen Race for the Cure®

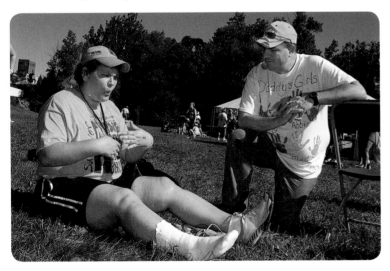

with a good friend, but the whole time, she says, she was "just overwhelmed by the urge to do the Breast Cancer 3-Day. When her friend agreed to do it with her, they signed up—with only two months left to train and raise money. "We didn't have any problem raising the money because people were so giving," says Jennifer, "but we definitely could have used a little more training."

At first, says Jennifer, her motivation was herself. "I walked so that I wouldn't have to worry so much about a recurrence, so that if or when I do have a recurrence all this money we raise might have helped find a cure." That soon changed. Two weeks into her training, Jennifer became friends with a couple who had started attending her church. The woman, Theresa, was 35, had two small children, and had been diagnosed with stage 4 breast cancer. "Her cancer had spread everywhere," says Jennifer, "and the tumors in her breasts were growing faster than they could shrink them. It just broke my heart. I kept asking, *Why is this happening? Why can't we find something to stop this?*" From that point on, Jennifer was walking for Theresa. "Through the walk itself, when I was in so much pain and didn't think I could take it anymore, I would just say her name—'Theresa, Theresa, I'm walking for Theresa'—because people like her are the ones who need it the most."

Jennifer says the event was the most amazing thing she's ever experienced. "Getting married was amazing," she says. "Having my children was amazing. But this

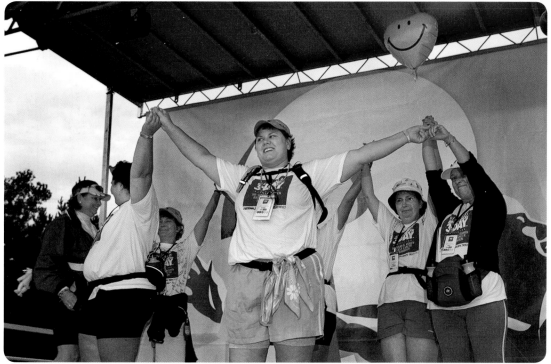

do the whole walk," says Jennifer. "In fact, he's walking regardless of what I do. So we're in a bit of a tug-of-war."

If there's one thing Jennifer hopes Jeff and her continued participation will accomplish, it will be to help dispel the myth that women under 40 and with no family history are not at risk. "I still have that lab report from when I was 26 that says, 'Follow with mammogram at age 40.' Hey," says Jennifer, "I wouldn't have made it to 40."

walk . . . it touched my soul to the deepest part. It was so wonderful." Reading all the journals in the Remembrance Tent was especially overwhelming. Her own entry read: "I walked for my four daughters—so that they may know breast cancer as something from the past, something they won't have to live in fear of."

Jennifer definitely plans to walk again, but first she wants to crew—"because if it weren't for those people, you wouldn't make it." Her husband, Jeff, who has been her rock of strength and support throughout her ordeal, has a different plan. He couldn't get away from work to do the entire walk with her the first time, but he managed to be there enough to catch the spirit. "Now he really wants to

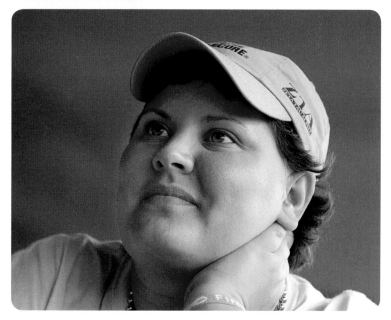

Tony Antoszewski

Chesterfield, Michigan

"When the fight against breast cancer came into our world, we embraced it so that maybe people in the future won't have to."

Tony Antoszewski remembers a day in the spring of 1998 when he and his bride-to-be, Sherrie, were registering for their wedding at Hudson's department store. A few days earlier Sherrie had had a surgical biopsy on a lump in her breast—"a simple procedure, local anesthetic"—and they had no reason to suspect that Sherrie's diagnosis would be anything other than the same sort of fibrous cysts her mother had had.

But the day before their trip to Hudson's, they'd gotten a call from the doctor's office reminding them of office policy: when coming in for the results of any surgical procedure, the patient had to bring a family member along with her. It wasn't hard for them to put two and two together.

"So there we were at Hudson's," says Tony, "practically throwing china at one another. We both knew we were

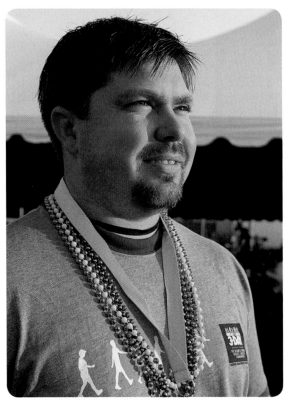

going to get this bad news the next day, but we just couldn't sit down and talk about it yet."

Sure enough, they got the bad news from a young oncologist who spared no detail. Sherrie would be bald for her wedding. And they could forget the honeymoon cruise because she would be on radiation and would need to stay out of the sun. "We absorbed it all," says Tony, "as well as a couple of 24-year-olds could."

Sherrie had a lumpectomy, and based on the size of the mass that was removed and the fact that the lymph nodes tested positive, she was diagnosed with stage 2. "That was a lot to deal with," says Tony, "but that was just Round One."

During Sherrie's last week of radiation therapy, she became pregnant—an event so improbable that she and Tony didn't realize it until some three months later. "We had been told that she would be at least temporarily sterile," says Tony,

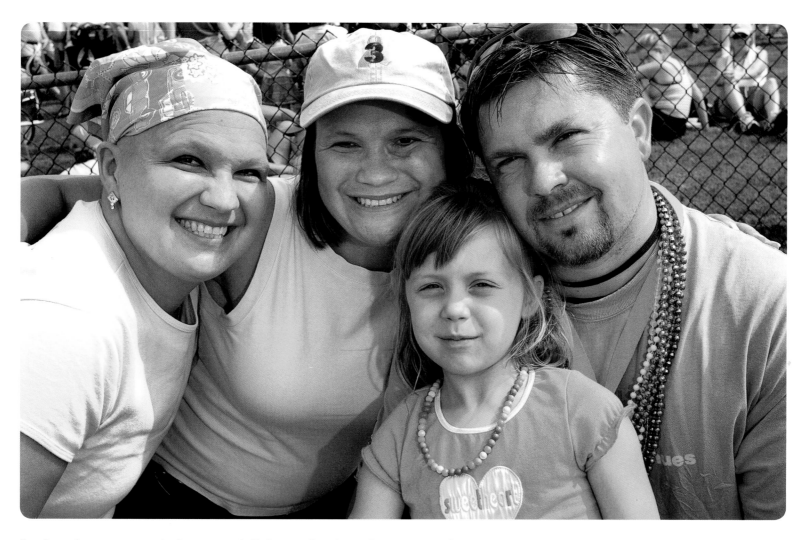

"and maybe permanently, because of all the medications she was taking." Nor were the doctors particularly pleased with this development. "They were telling us, frankly, that for Sherrie to have a healthy baby was highly unlikely."

That was an opinion they weren't prepared to accept from cancer specialists, so they visited what Tony calls "a high-risk ob-gyn." Tony says that as soon as they walked into the man's office, he knew that the news here would be good. "I'm a technology person," he says, "and I sensed that this technology was going to tell us that everything was okay with this baby." Tony was right. "The doctor told us that all the signs indicated that Sherrie was carrying a particularly healthy child." When Sherrie came to term, she delivered a perfectly healthy baby girl.

That happy occasion came in October 1999, but the next year Sherrie's cancer showed up in her other breast. She decided to have a complete mastectomy, and since she had recently given birth, she opted to have the surgeons use her abdominal tissue to reconstruct her breasts. Tony says he can't resist joking that his wife is the only woman he knows who got her health insurance "to pay for a tummy tuck and a boob job."

When Sherrie's cancer returned yet a third time 18 months later, she and Tony would need all the humor, fortitude, and sheer will they could muster. "We're thinking, *How can this possibly be?*" says Tony. "I mean, she's had both breasts removed. She's had chemo and radiation. Why is all this not killing the cancer?" In fact, the cancer had metastasized to Sherrie's lung, and her diagnosis was now stage 4. Unbelievably, the family had yet more terrible news to deal with. Sherrie's twin sister, Dawn, learned that she, too, had breast cancer.

At this point, in May 2002, you might think Tony and Sherrie would have just given up and crawled underneath the covers. Instead they decided to participate in a three-day breast cancer walk. "You don't hear many stories about people as young as Sherrie having breast cancer," says Tony. "We see what has happened to us as part of the education about the disease that people need to understand. Until you are touched by it," he continues, "it is not part of your world. Well, it has now become a major part of our world."

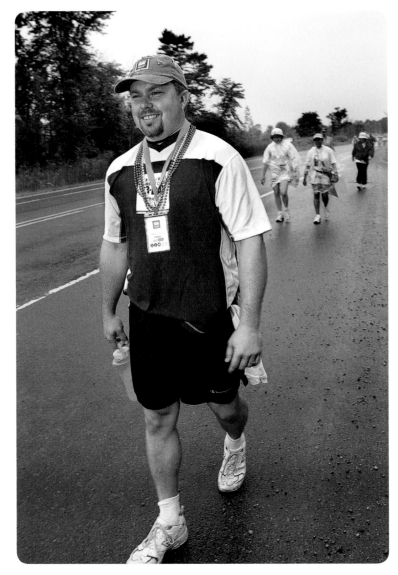

The walk was "a great experience," says Tony, and one they were looking forward to repeating when the Breast Cancer 3-Day came to Detroit in 2004. But with sister Dawn also hoping to participate, the fundraising became too much of an obstacle. Sherrie decided to simply stay with Dawn and let Tony do the walking, which he undertook with his typical gusto and enthusiasm.

The first time around, back in 2002, Tony and Sherrie "trained like you wouldn't believe," along with a huge team called the Wild Women Walkers. This time, though, he didn't train at all and was fully prepared to be "swept." As it turned out, he found himself walking beside a woman who was determined to make it, so he walked the whole way just to give her encouragement. In the evening, as it began to rain, he went around helping people who were having trouble setting up their tents. "Hey," he says, "I knew how to do it and a lot of people didn't. Why not make it easier on somebody else?"

Tony walked with a newspaper story about Sherrie and Dawn fixed onto his back, another part of the education he tries to help advance. "I liked people knowing that story," he says, but his purpose was larger. "I walked for my wife, my sister-in-law, my daughter, and all the other people that might be affected by this disease."

What's more, he and Sherrie have already registered for next year's event, where they plan to be crew members. Sherrie has also volunteered to be on the committee bringing the Komen Race for the Cure® to Detroit.

If Sherrie and Tony seem amazingly tireless for a couple who have taken as many hard knocks as they have, Tony has no trouble explaining their commitment. "It takes numbers," he says. "You've got to have numbers to raise that awareness, and we want to add to those numbers." He

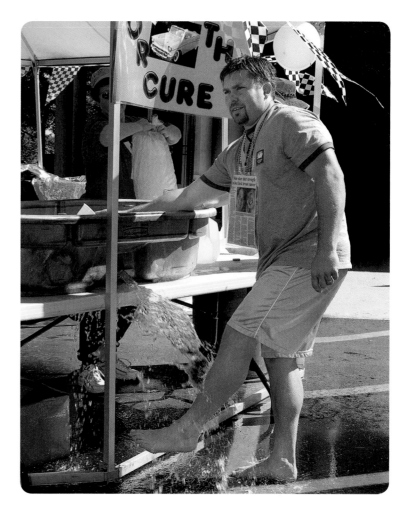

estimates that more than a thousand people now know about Sherrie's battle, "but if we all just sit at home and don't share our stories, then you'll never get those numbers of committed people."

Sherrie and Tony never planned to be in the front lines of the battle against breast cancer, but once the battle came to them, says Tony, "we embraced it—so that maybe in the future other people won't have to."

Jinx Vidrine

Mandeville, Louisiana

"We're going to raise money and find something every woman across the world can afford."

Some people just insist on turning catastrophe into catharsis. Jinx Vidrine was diagnosed in 1991 and finished her chemo in 1992. In 1993, she attended the Omega Institute, a holistic learning center founded in 1977 and located in Rhinebeck, New York. By then, she was already on the board of directors of "a little baby organization" called the Louisiana Breast Cancer Task Force. Her experience at Omega was so healing that she realized a similar resource was needed in her area.

When she brought the idea before the Task Force, the response was predictable: "We don't have any money for things like that." That wasn't about to stop her. "I did what the typical woman does," she says. "You beg every human being you know to pitch in: Would you cook food? Would you do a gumbo? Would you do this? Would you do that?" She pulled off an "almost free" retreat, charging only for the cost of housing.

Still, though, "a lot of the poor people couldn't come," and Jinx wanted to reach those people. "I thought, *I'll just sponsor it and make it free for everybody.*" Bad idea.

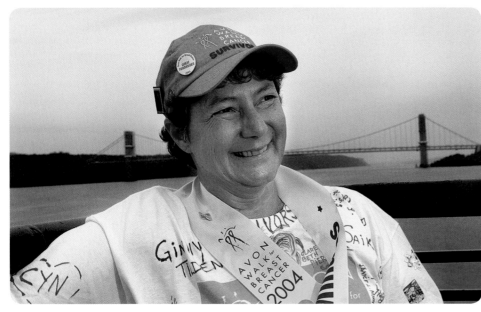

"Free was terrible. Everybody said, 'Yeah, yeah, I'm coming,' but since they hadn't put any money down they didn't show up." Finally she found the right formula: $50 for the whole weekend—just enough of a commitment so the people who say they're coming do in fact show up. And it's wonderful. The weekend starts with a wine and cheese reception the first evening—"to relax everybody and get them in the mood to talk." Then, going around in a circle, everybody tells their story and the bonding begins. Jinx uses a relaxation technique called Laughter: everybody

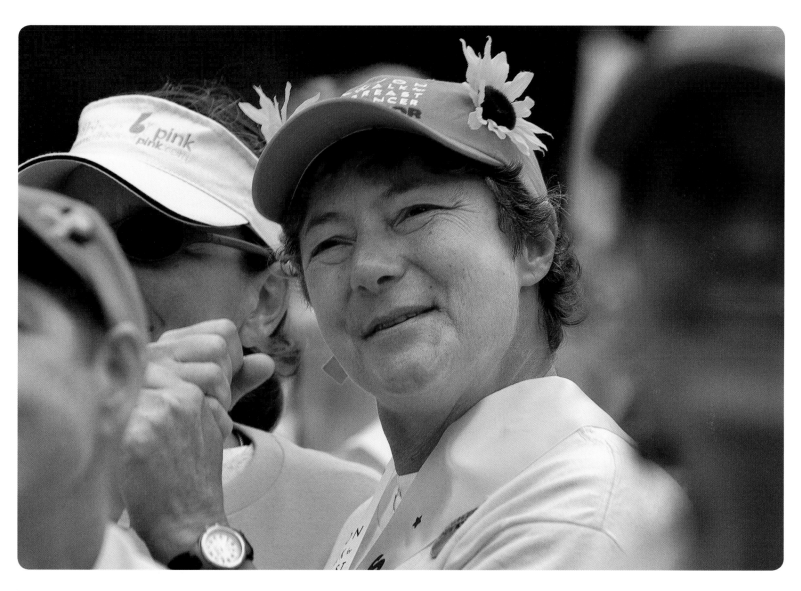

has to tell a joke or a funny story. Soon they're around the campfire, eating s'mores, giggling, opening up, sharing.

The goal of the retreat, says Jinx, is to face the question: okay, I've got cancer, what now? "We talk about fear. We set up goals. We ask, 'What are you dying to do that you haven't done?'" And it's at that point that the women "become magical among themselves." One might say, "I've always wanted to go to Paris," and another will jump in and say, "Okay, let's go." One wants to finish college, and another will show her how possible that is. "It happens

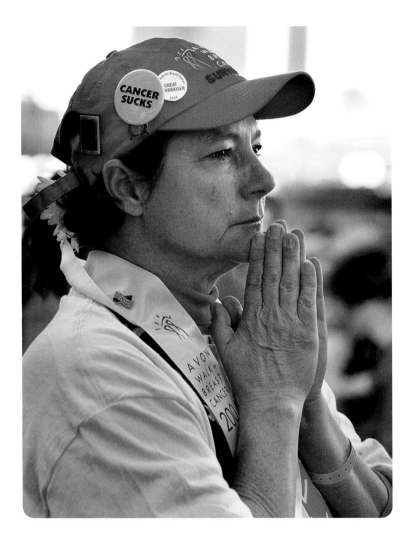

"and that word is *recurrence*." It was terrible—a half-hour of radiation every morning for six weeks. "I was so burnt," says Jinx, "I thought it was the garbage I was smelling."

Out of that experience, though, came Jinx's commitment to walking, raising money, and raising awareness. She saw an announcement for an Avon Walk in *Oprah* magazine and knew at once it was something she had to do. "I am going to raise money for something better than that mammogram," she told herself. "A blood test or saliva or urine. Something that all women can afford across the world." She sent a fundraising e-mail to everybody she knew: "I am tired of life challenging me," it read. "I'm going to pick my own challenge this year. Please support me in this walk."

Jinx signed up for the Avon Walk in San Francisco and started training: long three-and-a-half-hour walks in the early morning along a beautiful trail, "no phones, no distractions, just nature." Her first realization was what it was doing for her. "I go in for my checkup, and the doctor says, 'What are you doing? Look at these blood scores.'" Her cholesterol was down 28 points and her immune system was getting stronger for the first time in 10 years. "Training for that walk was working on me mentally, physically, and spiritually."

Then, on the walk itself, something else happened. Jinx saw a young woman with a picture of her mother on her backpack and a sign that said, "Keep fighting." The woman was crying and Jinx tried to comfort her. "I said,

every time," says Jinx, "and I'm always astounded. All of a sudden they're solving each other's problems." They beg to come back the next year, but Jinx has to tell them no—there are too many others who need the experience.

Jinx has been holding the retreat for 10 years now. The only year she missed was 2003, when her own cancer recurred. "There is a worse word than *cancer*," she says,

'Hey, it's okay.' I had my little "SURVIVOR" hat on." But the woman would not be consoled. She told Jinx that her mother had had a mastectomy three months before, but the cancer had spread into her lymph nodes and now there was no hope. Her mother was dying. "I looked at her and told her, 'Listen, it spread into my lymph nodes 12 years ago.'" Jinx says the woman fell down onto her knees sobbing—right in the middle of the walk. Then she tore into her backpack, pulled out a cell phone, called her mother, and said, "*Mom! Mom!* You're gonna live! Talk to this woman!"

"That's when I knew I had to keep walking," says Jinx. "Because at that moment in time, I represented hope." A few months later, Jinx walked in the Avon Foundation event in New York City. "Now," she says, "it looks like we're getting a team together to go to Chicago—the Bayou Blisters."

Jinx doesn't see herself as remarkable. "Everyone holds a treasure," she says, "but they just don't know how to use their gift." She believes that people would reach out—if only they knew what to do or how. "What's needed is a sense of community," says Jinx, "and that's exactly what you feel at these walks—that sense of belonging."

Allen Brown, Stacie (Brown) Heichel, Ryan & Fiona (Brown) Blanchard

Detroit, Michigan

"I was sore for a week, and I can't wait to do it again next year." —*Allen Brown*

Fiona "Mum" Brown must be very proud. This nine-year breast cancer survivor had already seen her three children demonstrate their love and support by participating regularly in the Komen Race for the Cure®. And when the Breast Cancer 3-Day came to Detroit, they were ready to walk those 60 miles. "I just had to mention it to my sisters," says her son Allen, "and they were on board right away."

According to Allen, this already-close family grew even closer during the three-day event. For the first time he and 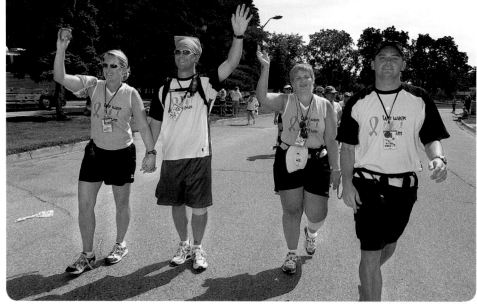 his siblings really talked about how their mother's sickness had affected their lives, how much they thought about it, how committed they have become to the battle against breast cancer. And in camp during the evenings, it looked like a Brown family reunion in progress, with parents, children, and grandchildren playing card games together or diving into daughter Fiona's birthday cake.

Even the T-shirts they walked in were a family affair. With son-in-law Ryan Blanchard joining the team, the slogan on the front of the shirt—"WE WALK 4 MUM"—carried a poignant double meaning. The pink ribbons festooning the front were computer-created by Stacie's daughters, six-year-old Courtney and five-year-old Haylie, while Allen, Stacie, and Fiona put their heads together to come up with the message of thanks printed on the back of the shirts: "WE ASKED, YOU GAVE, WE TRAINED, YOU CHEERED. WE WALK TO FIGHT BREAST CANCER." Ryan, an architect whom Allen calls the creative member of the family, pitched in on the overall design.

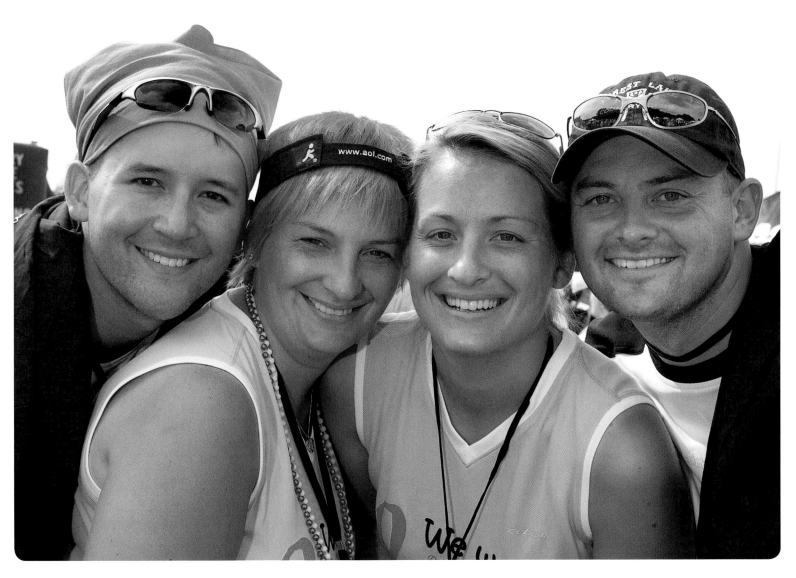

In fact, Allen says his brother-in-law's total involvement in the event is a testimony to two things. "First, it says what kind of person my mom is—just one of those people that, once you meet her, you can't forget her." Second, it says a lot about Ryan, who otherwise has no connection to breast cancer. "He just stepped in and has made this something very important in his life, as well," says Allen. "I think that's really impressive." But for Ryan, participation in the event offered its own great reward: "What I feel I accomplished," he says, "is knowing that when one day there is no such thing as breast cancer, I will have helped end this disease."

For Allen, the weekend's most memorable moment came at the closing ceremonies, when it was announced that the event had raised a staggering $4.4 million. "I think when it comes down to it," he explains, "the most important thing you need is money to fight the disease and find a cure, and it just boggles my mind to think that we raised so much money. That just the four of us could raise $10,000 was pretty amazing, too."

For Fiona, the event was "all about awareness" because she sees raising awareness as the direct route to saving lives. "Maybe someone driving down the street saw us all out there and decided to go get a mammogram, or donate money, or just talk about what they saw to someone else," says Fiona. "If just one person becomes more aware of breast cancer, I feel we've made a difference."

Stacie was astounded that such a huge number of people were willing to give their time—and their bodies—to the cause. "Until you have trained and walked those 60 miles," says Stacie, "it's pretty hard to imagine just how difficult it is—physically and mentally." Stacie also believes that such a huge commitment sends a powerful message. "If a single person who has been affected by breast cancer saw us on the news or in the newspaper and found hope

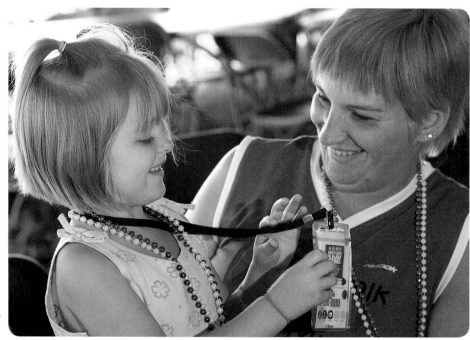

again, then we will have accomplished a great thing."

The team's plan was to start together and finish together but to be sure to interact with others along the way, and Allen says the people he met and the stories they told were an unforgettable part of the weekend. "There was a man walking with a shirt on that read, 'I MISS MY SIS,'" he recalls. "I spent just a few minutes talking to him, but I still haven't forgotten about him."

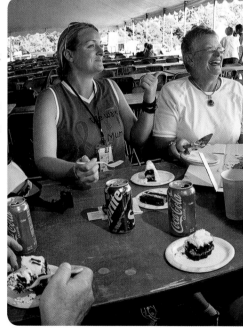

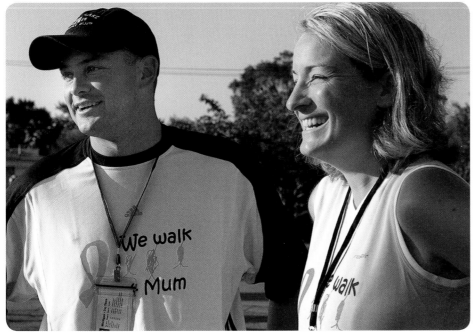

three-day span, I've never met so many people and *opened up* to so many people. You find yourself talking to complete strangers about very emotional feelings you might have had 10 years ago."

What's more, that sense of sharing and communication continues to spread outward after the event is over. "Having participated in the walk is a conversation starter," says Allen. "Talking about it back at work, for example, I learned for the first time my boss's connection to the disease. It's unbelievable how many people have been touched."

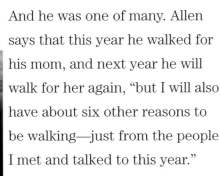

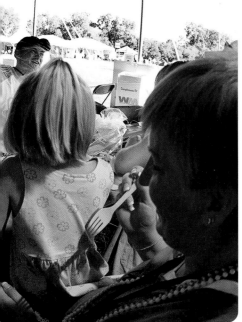

And he was one of many. Allen says that this year he walked for his mom, and next year he will walk for her again, "but I will also have about six other reasons to be walking—just from the people I met and talked to this year."

"It's amazing how you build a community," continues Allen. On Friday, a few thousand people come together for a common purpose. By Sunday, they've become a community of friends and soulmates. "Over a

As remarkable as anything else, says Allen, is the spirit of good will, of celebration, even of joy that prevailed for the entire weekend. And it's all the more remarkable given the physical pain of the grueling 60-mile walk. "I had parts of my body hurt those three days that I didn't even know could hurt, but I got up in a great mood every morning." And then there were all the "awesome support people, lining the route even in the rain, handing out candy and apples, cheering us on."

Allen says it's not easy to explain to somebody who hasn't done it that walking 60 miles can be such an inspiring and spirit-lifting experience. "All I know is I was sore for a week, and I can't wait to do it again next year."

Walking to
Raise Awareness

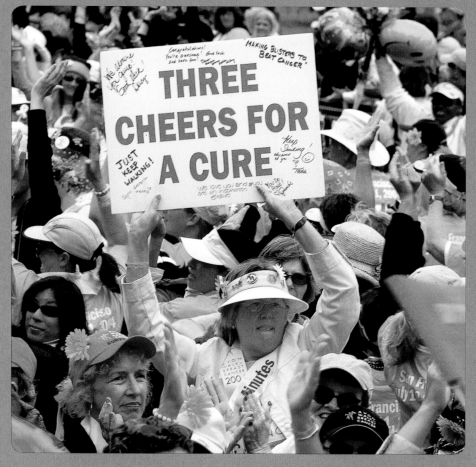

THREE CHEERS FOR A CURE

The terrible fact is that every three minutes a woman is diagnosed with breast cancer in the United States. A more hopeful truth is that early detection saves lives. These walks promote early detection by providing an opportunity to educate and inform the public about breast cancer and create awareness on a grassroots level. Walkers reach out to their friends, family, and community to ask for their support in fundraising and training efforts. Whether the event is 5 miles, 40 miles, or 60 miles, every step makes a difference in the fight against breast cancer.

I walk because...

"Each step is definitive progress toward eliminating cancer ... saving loved ones and keeping families and friends intact rather than painful memories. I walk for my mom ... one of the many lovely and beautiful moms that have been taken from us way too early." —*Mike Kelly*

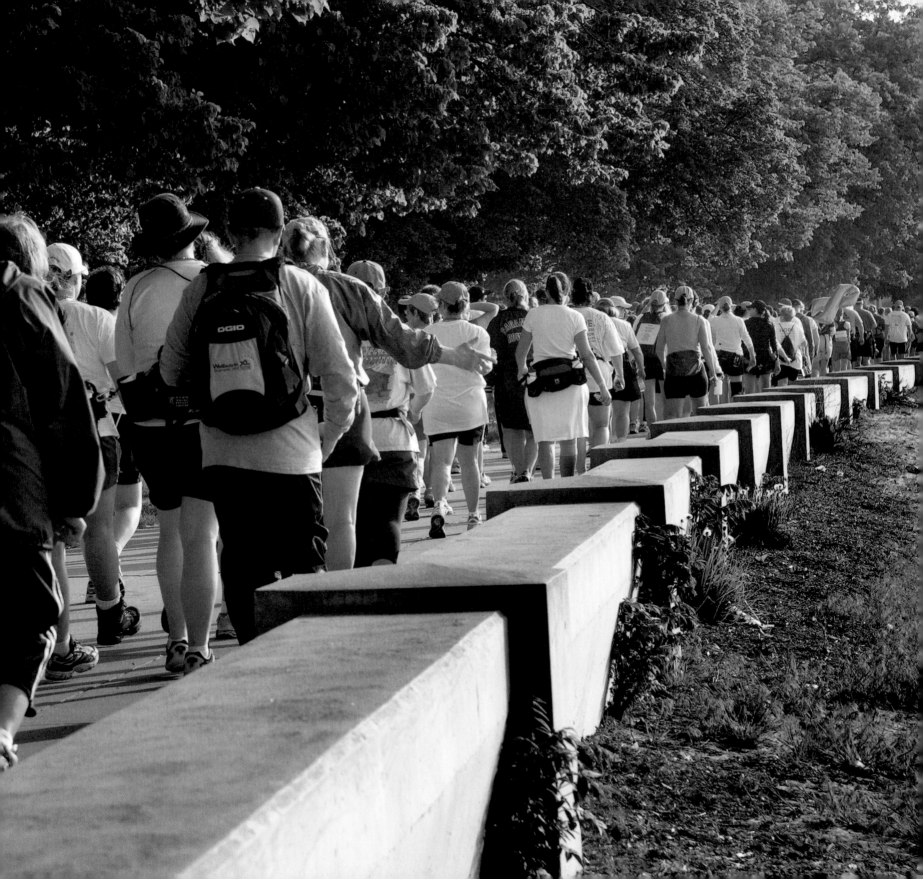

Paul Boulanger & Men With Heart

Boston, Massachusetts

"We're not looking for attention. We want to give attention."—Paul Boulanger

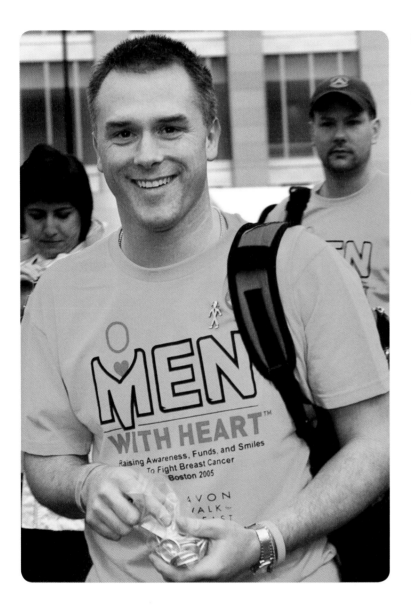

When Paul Boulanger signed up to participate in the Avon Breast Cancer 3-Day in Boston in 2001, he was in for two surprises. First was what an incredibly rewarding experience it was. Second was the fact that of some 3,000 participants, only 88 were men.

"I thought that was a terrible statistic," says Paul, whose wife at the time had just been diagnosed. "While it's true that the disease most often affects women's bodies, there's almost an equal number of men directly involved in those women's lives." But it wasn't just that the event was missing out on male participation; men were missing out on an incredible experience. "It's such an uplifting event," says Paul. "The camaraderie, the bonding, the emotional ties, the stories, the laughs, the tears—I just couldn't believe that more men didn't want to take part in something like that."

Paul decided to do something "to get men involved" in the fight against breast cancer, so for the 2002 Avon Walk he persuaded 36 of his friends to walk with him, and Men With Heart was born. "We raised $135,000 at that one event," says Paul. Not surprisingly, it was the largest organized group of men in the Avon Walk's history.

But for this big-hearted group, walking and raising money is not enough. As the organization's Web site puts

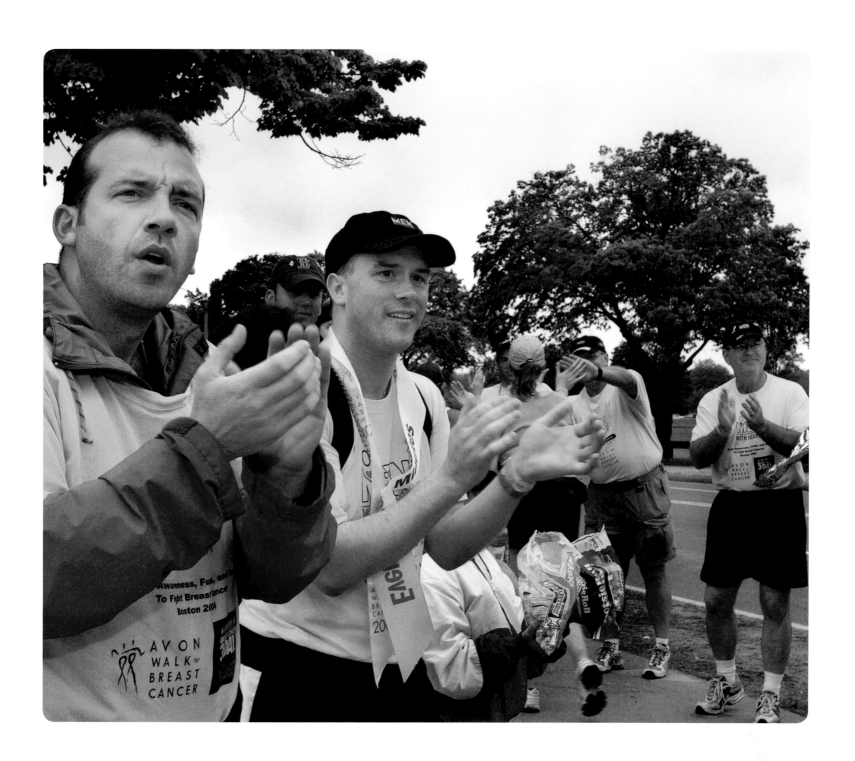

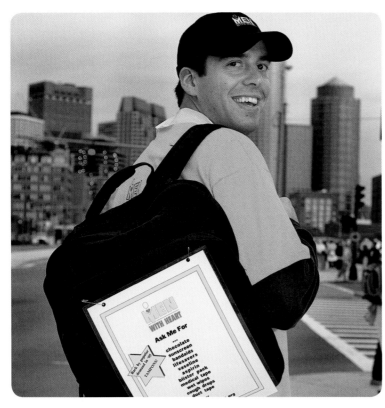

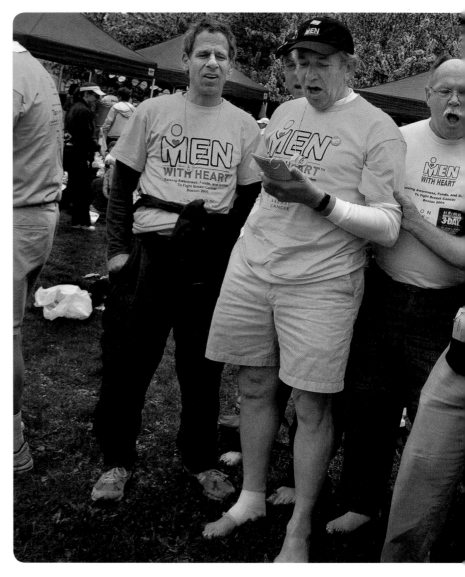

it, their goal is "to raise awareness, funds, and smiles." Wearing their signature yellow T-shirts, the men sing songs, cheer, and do whatever it takes to revive flagging spirits. Also, what began with one of the guys toting a backpack with candy has evolved into an integral part of the group's image and mission. Now all team members carry "MEN WITH HEART" backpacks loaded with supplies—not just sweets, but also sunscreen, blister packs, clean socks, and even tampons. Each pack bears a list of its inventory and a sign that reads, "ASK ME FOR . . ."

As founding member Scott Walters explains, "We're just trying to figure out the best way to be cheerleaders and to lend support. We're there to help, and Rule One is that none of the guys are allowed to complain."

"We decided to have fun with it," adds Paul, "to make sure everybody has a good time. We're not looking for attention. We want to give attention."

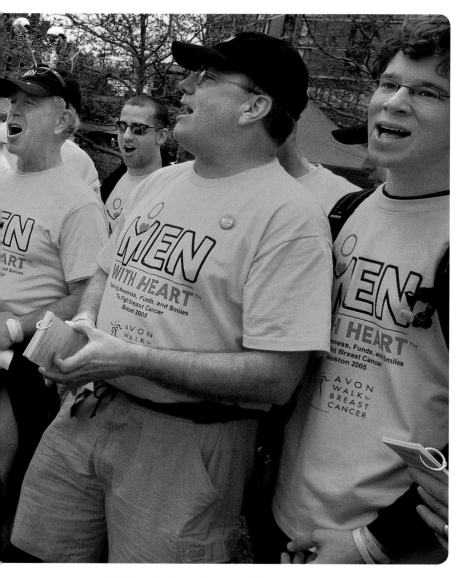

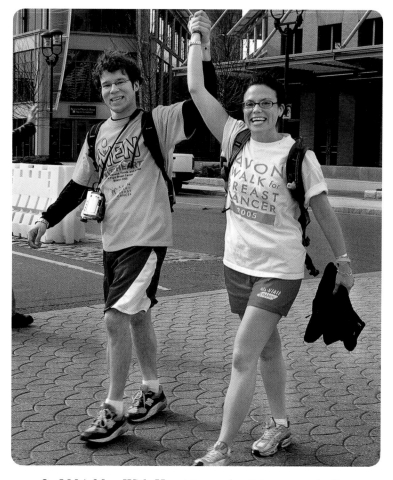

In 2004, Men With Heart turned out to support all three major breast cancer events in Boston—including the Avon Walk, the Breast Cancer 3-Day benefiting the Susan G. Komen Foundation, and the American Cancer Society's Making Strides Walk. Today, Men With Heart is an accredited 501(c)(3) public charity, and it has contributed more than $300,000 for breast cancer–related causes.

What do he and his group get out of giving? "At the end of the 2002 event," says Paul, "our group gathered

Making it fun makes good sense, too. Paul points out that if the women participants enjoy the event enough, next year they'll bring along their husbands, fathers, brothers, sons, and friends. Which will mean yet more awareness, more support, and more financial contributions, to this worthy cause.

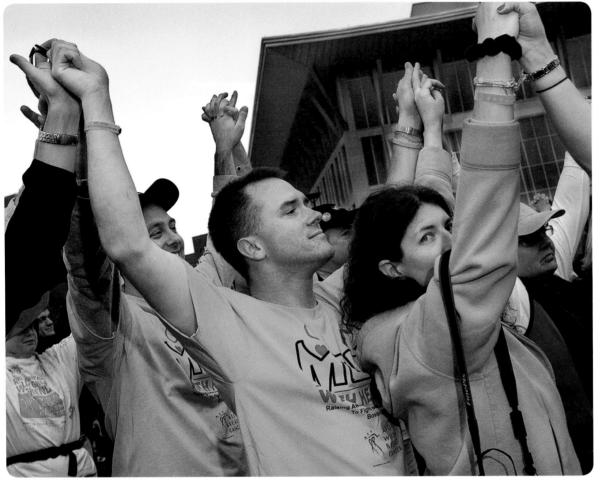

most amazing emotional experience any of us have ever had. We get way more out of the event than we put in."

But based on the e-mails that pour into the group's Web site from grateful walkers, Men With Heart "puts in" quite a lot. In fact, in November 2004 Paul was awarded the Avon Foundation's Community Advocacy Award at the annual Kiss Goodbye to Breast Cancer Award Celebration in New York City—in recognition of Men With Heart's "extraordinary effective-

at the end of the Massachusetts Avenue Bridge about an hour and a half before the closing ceremony so that we could cheer everybody on as they came across the bridge. That meant that we were among the last walkers into the Government Center Plaza, and when we walked in, we got a standing ovation from the 3,000-plus people gathered there. The reception we got—the appreciation—was so incredible that all of us men had tears in our eyes. It was the

ness and mission to involve men in the breast cancer cause." Paul says it was "an incredible honor—to be in the company of people like Ann Curry, news anchor for NBC News and Jonathon Simon, a world-famous physician who's leading the fight against breast cancer. It was really the experience of a lifetime."

That "mission to involve men" remains the group's driving purpose. In October 2004, Men With Heart staged its first annual Run With Heart 5K Race/Walk in Boston, an event Paul says was intended to raise money, awareness, *and* membership. "Just three new members means an additional $6,000 at the next breast cancer event," he says, "so we're building traction for the future."

Their work remains vital, as Scott puts it, because too many men are still "ostriches with their heads in the sand" when it comes to breast cancer. He himself was typical. His mother is now a 10-year survivor, but before he joined Paul in 2002, he says he was "clueless." He doubts that his father "really understood" what his mother was going through, either. "We need to have a better idea about this," he says. "We need to understand how pervasive and devastating this disease is."

Thus the group's eloquent definition of what Men With Heart is all about: "We are husbands who are doing

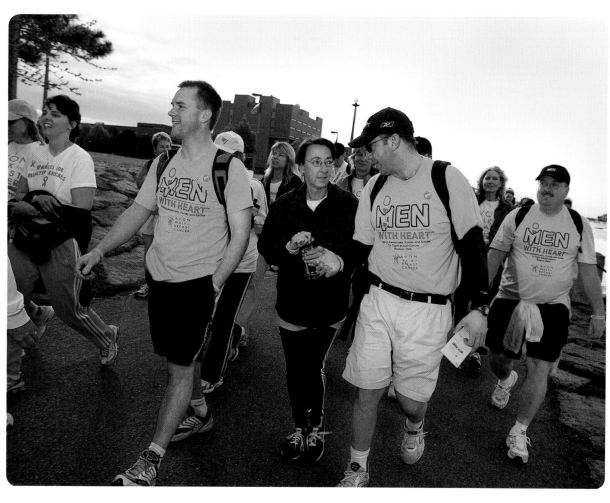

something constructive rather than resigning themselves to helplessness. We are sons who have seen their mothers courageously fight an insidious disease. We are brothers who want to stand beside our sisters in this battle. We are relatives, friends, lovers, colleagues, neighbors, and admirers of the women who are struggling with, often beating, and, regrettably, sometimes losing, the fight with breast cancer."

Vicky King

Rockville, Maryland

"I'm starting to think that sleep is terribly overrated. Either that or I've just gone insane."

Vicky King has four children and two jobs. What she doesn't have is time. But that didn't stop her from spending all summer training and then walking in the Breast Cancer 3-Day Walk in Washington, D.C.

She walked, she says, because her mother, her aunt, and her cousin were all diagnosed with breast cancer within the past year. She also had another aunt who died some years ago from what started out as breast cancer, "and I had to explain to my then 10-year-old what it means to have breast cancer in the family. I don't ever want to have to explain that to my grandchildren."

Vicky admits that she needed all the motivation she could get. A 60-mile walk is not generally her idea of a good time. Her husband and children were hedging their bets. "They saw everything involved—the training, the fundraising, plus everything else I have going on—and they were going, 'No way. She'll never do it.'" Plus, Vicky is not, in her words, "an athletic person." Not that she's lazy. "I don't sit on the sofa eating bonbons and watching soap operas all day," she says. "But my idea of exercise is walking to the freezer."

The fundraising was particularly difficult, and also unbelievably rewarding. She works two jobs to pay the bills, she says, not to hang out at the country club. She doesn't have rich friends "who can put in $100 or $200 or $500," so most of her donations were very small. "It was whatever they could afford, and I was grateful," says Vicky. "Honestly, the lady at church who gave me the 60¢ meant as much to me as the lady at church who gave me my one big $150 donation. Actually, it meant more because that 60¢ was probably every cent she had in her purse."

Then there was the 20-year-old kid at work, "a young male—nobody he knows personally or is close to has been diagnosed." But one night after work this young man came in and handed Vicky $75. "'Hey,' he says, 'my friends and I have been raising this for you.' His only motivation was that he saw what I was trying to do and he and his friends wanted to help."

As for the walk itself, Vicky says she was "totally impressed" by everybody that turned out—the walkers, the crew, the staff, the volunteers, "even the people who stopped to cheer and honk and wave." She loved "the camaraderie that developed, how everybody just kind of pulled together." On the whole, though, Vicky believes that the crew and the volunteers deserve the most credit. "They don't get the glory that the walkers get," she says, "but they're out there working just as hard, if not harder. You know, we can always say, 'Enough's enough, I can't

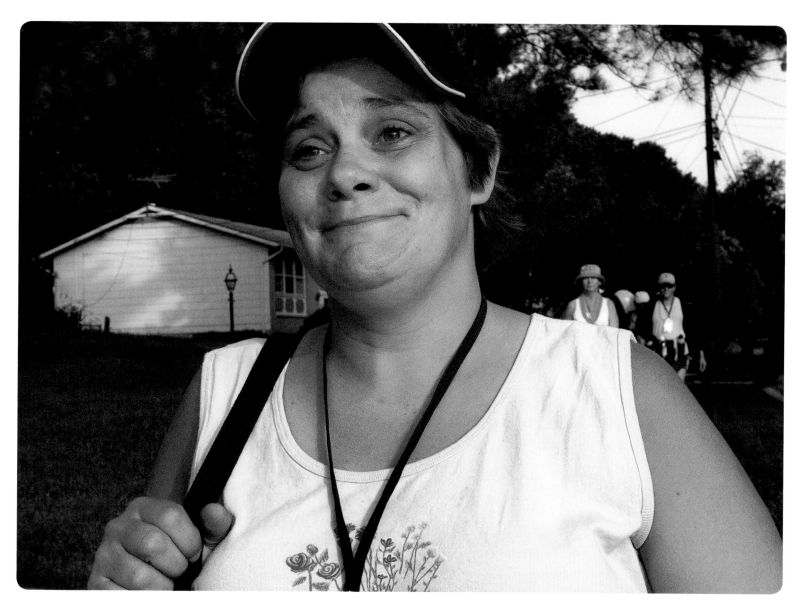

walk any farther,' and jump on the bus out of there. But they're still out there directing traffic, standing in the rain, doing all the things that have to be done—even after we're all safe and snug and dry."

Vicky was also surprised, even shocked, by all the attention lavished on her personally. She was walking by herself, not partnered with anybody, not on anybody's team, but still, she says, "All these people were watching out for me."

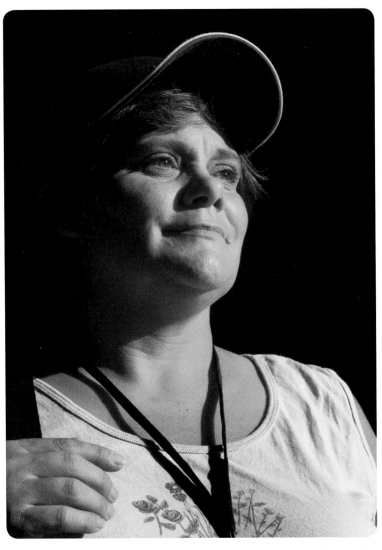

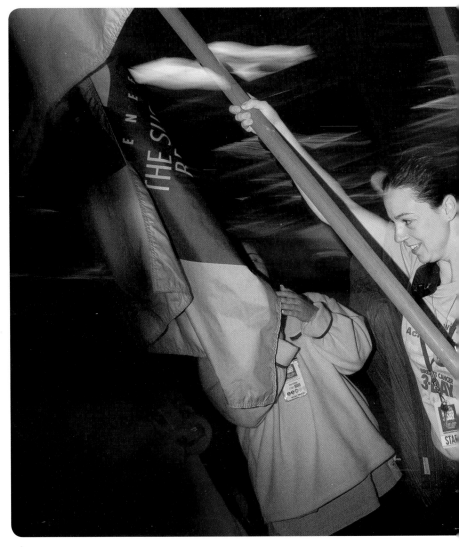

The outpouring of support was magnified on Saturday evening when Vicky was the last walker home. Walkers usually spend Saturday night in a "tent city," but remnants of the recent hurricanes had forced the spend-the-night to move inside the Expo Center. As the last walker in, it was Vicky's honor to carry the flag, and she found herself walking down a long aisle lined on both sides by throngs of wildly cheering participants.

"I was totally mortified," she recalls with a laugh. "I'm not one to be in the spotlight, and all day long I kept saying to myself, *I'm not going to be the last walker in. I'm not going to have everybody looking at me.*" In photographs,

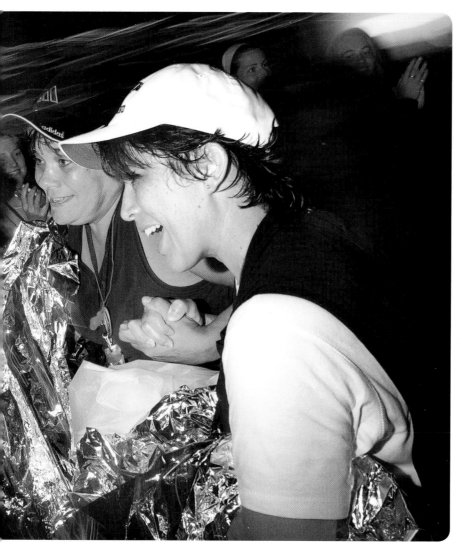

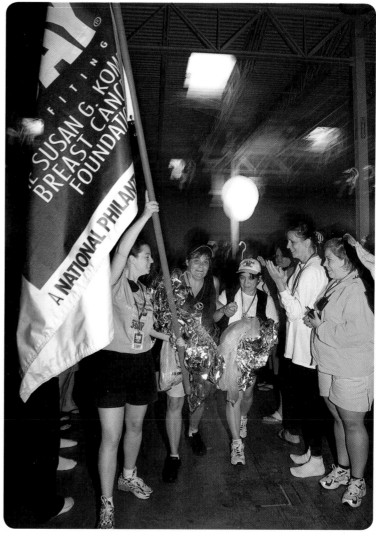

says Vicky, she's the one hiding in the back. During her year as PTA president, if you gave her three minutes to say what she needed to say, you would have one left over.

So picture Vicky walking those final steps down the aisle inside the center, with all the walkers inside yelling and clapping. "It really was just amazing."

Vicky's only regret is that because of the plantar fasciitis that troubles her feet, she has to give up the idea of walking in another event. But she says she would jump at the chance to be a volunteer or crew member. "The Komen Foundation is doing a wonderful job," she says, "and I would love to be able to help in the future."

Susan Jones

Accokeek, Maryland

"Never give up. Do everything you can now. And don't let a day or an hour or a minute go by wasted."

In the aftermath of the Breast Cancer 3-Day Walk in Washington, D.C., the first thing Susan Jones wanted to talk about was her mother. When she staggered into camp after the first day's 20 miles, "*soooo* tired and every bone hurting," her mother had the tent set up and everything all laid out—even though, says Susan, "My mother is not exactly a camp person." Best of all was the desperately needed, lovingly administered foot massage.

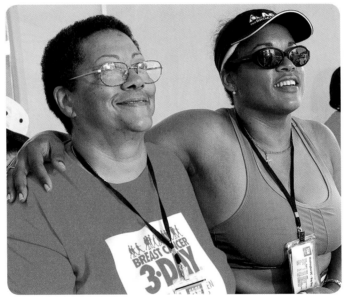

"When you're tired and achy and pitiful, you want your mom—no matter how old you are," says Susan. If she hadn't had her mother waiting, she's sure she wouldn't have made it. "They would have had to pick me up somewhere on the parkway, just lying on the side of the road, like a deer that had been hit in the middle of the night."

Don't be fooled by the apparent faintheartedness. When Susan explains how her mom happened to be there, you begin to understand a little more about Susan herself.

"Mom is 62 years old," says Susan, "arthritic, bad back, you name it, and she's still working. As the time for the walk came closer and closer and she got involved with helping me fundraise, she said, 'Okay, when is it? I'm coming, too.' I told her she wasn't walking any 60 miles, and she said, 'Well, then, find out what I can do to volunteer.' When I told her they needed medical people, she said, 'That'll work. I'm trained for that.'"

Susan doesn't fit the profile of the breast cancer walker. She's not a survivor, nor was she walking on behalf of a friend or loved one. She's a very busy full-time mother with four kids at home, ages 3 to 14. But make no mistake. The battle against breast cancer is fortunate to have fearless soldiers like Susan in its ranks.

Her mission as a participant is clear-cut: to support the effort to find a cure. She's not sure that the medical/pharmaceutical community always has its priorities

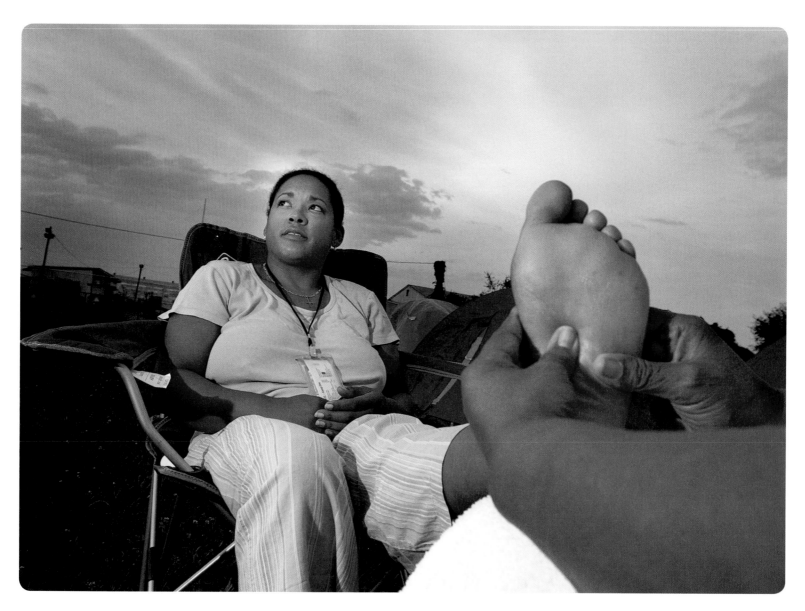

in order, and she doesn't mind saying so: "I'm walking for anybody who has to suffer from this disease. I mean, it irritates me that in a matter of a few years we could find several drugs to combat impotence in males, but we can't cure breast cancer? I know it's not the easiest thing to get rid of, but does that mean we should limit funding to the things that we *can* get rid of? If that was the case, we'd still be walking around with polio."

Moreover, as a Black woman who's well aware of breast cancer's higher mortality among her own population, she has a secondary mission: to get her sisters in the African-American community to come to their senses. "We've had all these problems for generations—diabetes and heart problems and obesity and poor diet, and I still see a great number of African-American women who don't exercise because

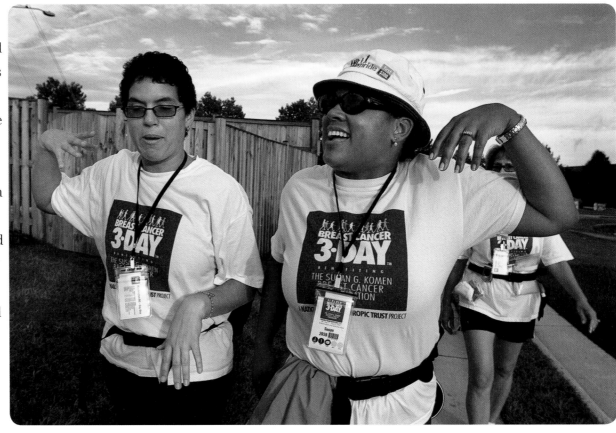

they don't want to mess up their hair! It's ludicrous. And when it comes to breast cancer, these women say they don't get mammograms because it hurts! I'm like, *Are you nuts?* If you think a mammogram hurts, how do you think chemo feels?"

Susan admits that with all her responsibilities at home, it wasn't easy to give three days to a breast cancer walk, to say nothing of the many other days she spent training for the event. But she says she was simply doing what she tries to teach her children to do: "If you want to

change something, if you are not satisfied with how something is going, you're going to have to get off your duff and do something about it."

Susan is no stranger to the battlefield. The younger of her two sons, aged nine, is blind. As of last year, she says, he had undergone close to 63 eye surgeries. "I have had my fill of physicians telling me, 'This is all we can do.' I tell them, 'You mean, this is all you are *interested* in doing.' I tell them, 'Have you looked in the Yellow Pages under physicians? You're not the only one in the book.'"

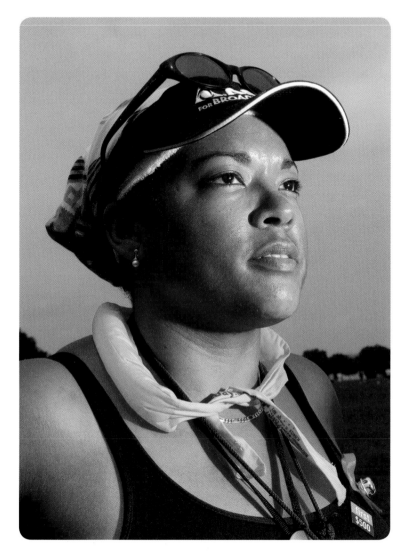

Nobody has to remind Susan that bad things happen, but her experience has taught her that people don't need pity. "You may need comforting, yes. You may need a friend. Definitely you want information, assistance, and treatment. But you don't want pity. And you don't want negativity. The last thing you want is somebody telling you that this is the best you can do."

Susan says that, regrettably, her days as a cancer walker are over. She has just found out that, like her mother, she has osteoarthritis. "The doctor tells me my hip is like that of a 62-year-old woman's. He's talking about replacement surgery."

Somehow it seems unlikely that an arthritic hip will slow down Susan Jones, who confesses that the two words that best describe her are *perseverance* and *dedication*. If she's not walking, you can bet she'll be talking, and her message will be loud and clear.

There is an analogy between what her son has been through and what many women experience after they've been diagnosed, and Susan can't stand the thought of settling for anything less than all that is possible. "For every 5 people who are going to tell you no," she says, "there are 150 waiting to tell you yes."

Sandy & Jack Jordan

Chicago, Illinois

"A big piece of the puzzle of my life has fallen into place." —*Sandy Jordan*

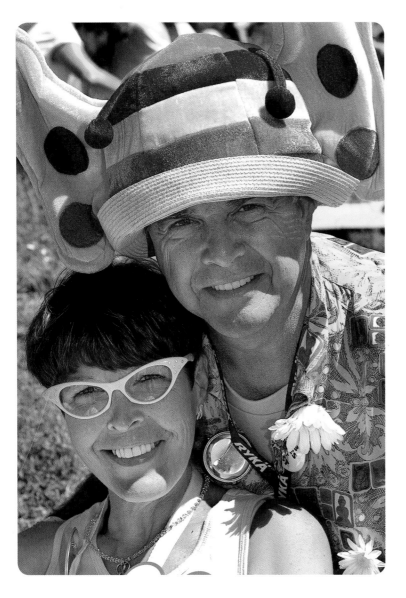

Sandy Jordan doesn't mind admitting that she has "fought weight" all of her life. When the Avon Breast Cancer 3-Day came to Chicago in 2000, she was inspired. "I saw so many sizes, so many types, women and men out there. I said to myself, *If they can do it, so can I*. I told Jack [her husband] I wanted to do that the next year, and he was like, 'Yeah, right.'"

Sandy had already decided to have gastric bypass surgery in January 2001. "Four hours out of surgery," she says, "Jack started walking with me, and he kept at it until I could walk on my own." When the Avon event came to town in June, Sandy had lost 157 pounds. Walking the 60 miles that weekend was a "real accomplishment."

The thing about those real accomplishments, though, is that they make you want more. "The whole thing just addicted me," she says. "Not just the physical challenge, but also the wonderful people that you meet." In 2002, Sandy walked in Chicago again and also in San Francisco, but that was like giving a drop of water to a woman dying of thirst. She decided that in 2003 she would walk in all eight Avon Walk for Breast Cancer events.

But how? Sandy cleans houses for a living. Jack is a fireman. Raising the money to register for eight events was

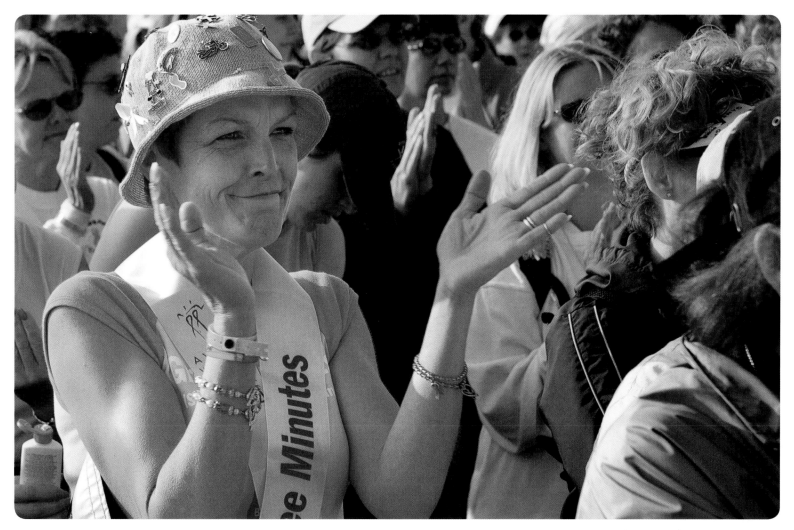

not going to be a simple matter of writing a check. What was more, taking the time to train for, travel to, and participate in every event meant that Sandy would have to give up half her clients—half her income. As she puts it, "The decisions I was making had a lot more to do with what filled my heart than what filled my pocket." Ultimately, says Sandy, the financial sacrifice wasn't that big a deal. All

they've had to give up is their vacations. From vacations you have pictures, says Sandy. You have memories. "But no vacation could ever take the place of the memories these last three years of my life have given me."

One of those special memories is of two survivors, Roberta and Gayle, whom Sandy met on her first walk in 2001. Walking with these two women, says Sandy, and imagining their young children having to grow up with-out their moms, was the experience that changed her life. "That's what really made me climb aboard," she says. "They were about my age, and the idea that I had an op-portunity to help them . . . well, they put a very big mark on my heart. It seemed like a big piece of the puzzle of my life was falling into place."

Another of Sandy's memorable encounters was with Mona, a "little lady with absolutely no hair" she met in New York in 2003. During the seven or eight miles they walked together, Mona told Sandy about being a two-time survivor "and everything that goes with that." Because Sandy was walking in every event, she was up on the stage during clos-ing ceremonies and saw Mona blow her a kiss from down on the ground. But when Sandy came down afterward and looked for her, Mona was nowhere to be found. Then, in San Francisco in 2004, "a woman walks up to me and says, 'Sandy?' I'm like, *Oh my God, it's Mona!* She's in complete remission, full head of hair, and ready to see her only son get married. It was so good. It was unbelievable."

But that wasn't the end of the story. Later in 2004, back in New York, Mona and her husband, Gary, tracked Sandy, Jack, and their son, Eric, down at their hotel and took them out to dinner. "It was so amazing," says Sandy. "I'm sure my dinner cost more than my weekly grocery bill. They treated my family like royalty. I had no idea. These people were billionaires." Here was another pro-found lesson to be learned from the breast cancer crusade.

As Sandy said to Mona's husband, "When you take away the diamonds and all the other stuff, you see that we're all on the same page in life." Gary knew just what she meant. "Yeah," he said. "What good is it to have everything in the world and not be able to save your wife?" An expensive meal in New York is a fine memory in itself, but to have Mona still in contact, by phone and e-mail, to tell Sandy how much she has meant, how she inspired Mona to make it another year, or just to say "thinking of you," well, "that puts a mark on your heart."

Still, when Sandy talks about the people that have meant the most to her throughout her involvement with the Avon Breast Cancer Crusade, her husband Jack stands first and foremost. When Sandy participated in every 2003 event, she "flew solo" because she had never done anything by herself before and that was part of the challenge. But when she wanted to do every event again in 2004, she couldn't hold him off any longer. He "jumped on the bandwagon" and crewed every event she walked in. "How he came aboard and adopted this cause that has meant so much to me will always hold a special place in my heart," says Sandy. "Honestly, we're not able to do this financially, but somehow, some way, my husband always makes it work."

What's more, Jack, whom Sandy describes as "always the macho fireman," does it just as joyfully and whole-heartedly as Sandy. "I picture him in black jeans and a Harley T-shirt. But here he is in a pink shirt, a wig, a dress—crying." Jack is always at the closing, his hand

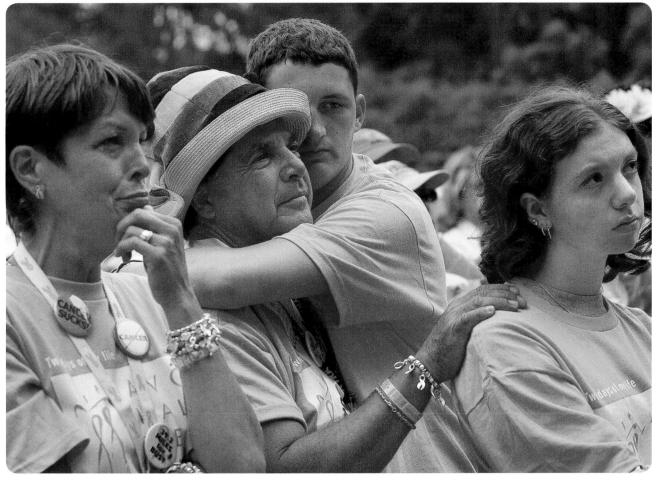

inspirational," he says, "I was like, *Oh my God, I've got to do something for this cause. I've got to get out there.*" Now, after crewing for a year, he says, only half-joking, that the walkers have it easy. But crewing offers its own special reward. "When the walkers thank me for making them feel good," says Jack, "that makes me feel good."

on hers, just so she will know he is there. "Yet he gave me every inch of the space that I needed to be able to fulfill my dream."

In fact, before crewing for the 2004 season, Jack walked with Sandy during the final 40-mile Avon Walk in 2003. "Sandy told me I couldn't do it," he recalls, "so of course I had to prove that I could." He was "addicted" as quickly as his wife. "Just the opening ceremony is so

Sandy and Jack's son, Eric, has joined the crusade, too. At 16, he's too young to crew, so he volunteers. "He says tough guys wear pink," reports Sandy.

As Jack sums up the experience, "People come up and say, 'Wow, your whole family is doing this stuff and the disease hasn't even affected you.' I say, 'Yes, it has. Maybe not directly, but it affects us indirectly because everybody here is our family now.'"

George Nummer

Clawson, Michigan

"It's like you're in another world out there. Everybody is so . . . well, everybody is just how you want people to be."

G ot problems? Feeling blue? Depressed? George Nummer has the solution for you: walk 60 miles for someone else's sake.

George's own depression settled in after he took off his electrician's tool belt for the last time. "I always thought working was a part of life, so I retired late," he says. "But even so, I felt at a loss." He and his wife had been living in California, and they moved back home to

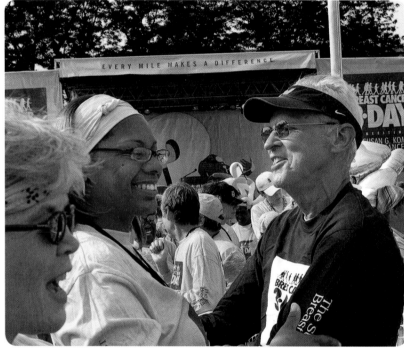

Michigan, into the house they had been renting out. It was in bad shape, but that was a good thing. It gave George something to do, but not enough. He still felt blue.

Then came September 11, 2001. "That really got me down," he says. "I was just very depressed, but then I heard President Bush say in one of his speeches that one way to fight terrorism was to help people. Help your neighbor. Get out and do something." Shortly thereafter,

he saw an announcement for a breast cancer walk that Avon was sponsoring. "I got the information and read the statistics and everything, and I just said, 'Boy, somebody has to do something about this.'"

So George, then 70 years of age, participated in the Avon event in 2002. He saw it as a way to help his country, to help others. What he didn't see was what it would do for him. "I really didn't realize how rewarding it would be, but after I got into it, it was like . . . it changed my whole life."

If Avon had sponsored another walk in Detroit in 2003, George would have been there. As it was, he was chomping at the bit when the Komen Foundation brought its Breast Cancer 3-Day to Detroit in 2004. He raised funds tirelessly and trained for months, working his way up to 12 miles a day, six days a week. His preferred routine was

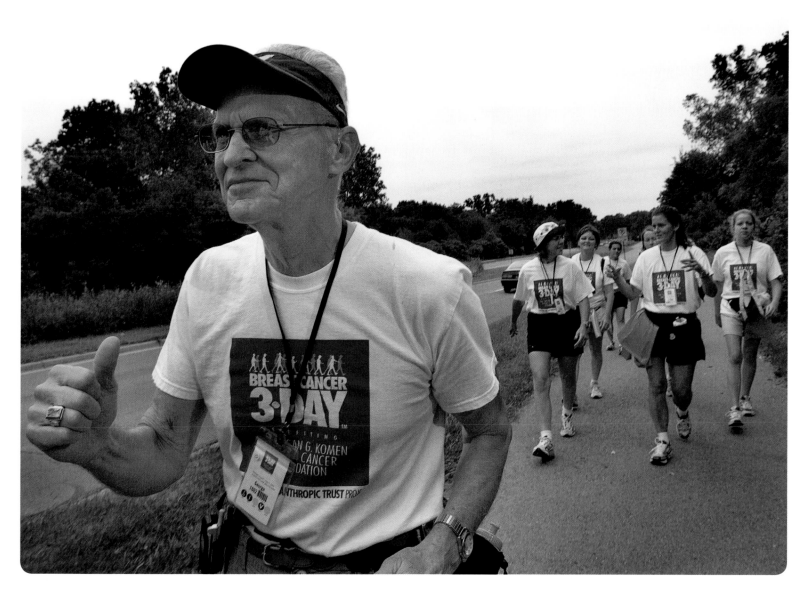

to get up at four in the morning and walk for two or three hours "when there's no traffic or exhaust fumes." Then he would come home and go back to bed for a couple of hours "and wake up fresh as a daisy."

In the last weeks leading up to the event, he cut back on his training miles to rest his feet. He knew he couldn't walk 60 miles without a few aches and pains, but, says George, "that's a small price to pay to help save even one life."

The Breast Cancer 3-Day was everything he thought it would be—and more. He was asked to help raise the flag at the closing ceremonies. "What a joy that was," George exclaims. "It just made the whole thing. It's hard to explain the feelings that you get out of something like that."

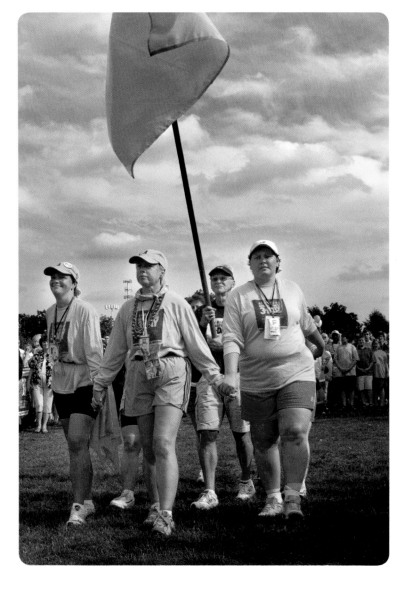

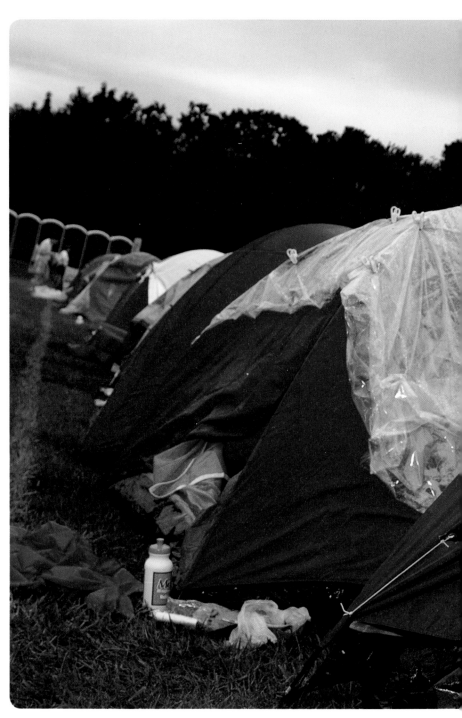

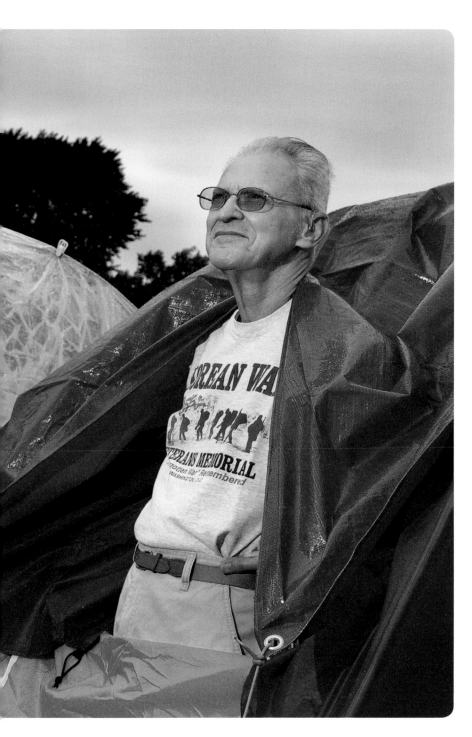

People were surprised to see a 72-year-old participant. What surprised George were the survivors he found himself walking with. "Those women have really got guts," he says admiringly. "Some of them didn't even have time to train. They're out there walking with blisters on their feet, their feet bleeding, and they just kept going for the cause. That was such a great inspiration to me."

George says that his own family has not been touched by breast cancer. For this man, that's just another reason to walk. "We've been very fortunate, and this is my way of thanking God." It's also his way of helping others, which is his way of helping himself. "We're all one," he explains. "I just get more joy out of helping others than I do out of thinking about myself."

No wonder, then, that George is already gearing up for 2005. He's even discovered a unique fundraising angle. He's been putting that tool belt back on, after all, and "taking a few jobs on the side." He charges only for materials, though; all money for his labor goes to fight breast cancer. He has even arranged things so that what his customers pay him for his work is tax deductible.

He also hopes to put together a fundraising support group. "Not everyone has time to participate in the race," he says, "but they still might want to help raise money. I'll do the walking and they can do the talking."

Walk on, George.

Camaraderie

These days, it's hard to imagine a world where everyone is united in a common cause, but that's exactly what happens at these events. The walls that separate us in everyday life have suddenly come down. Every walker commits to walking the distance through rain or shine, to sleeping in a tent city with portable toilets and mobile showers, and it's impossible not to make new friends along the way. Walkers talking, sharing stories, forming bonds that might last the weekend or a lifetime, everyone looking out for everyone else. "Are you okay? Need a shoulder to lean on?"

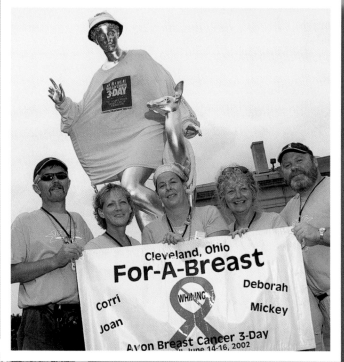

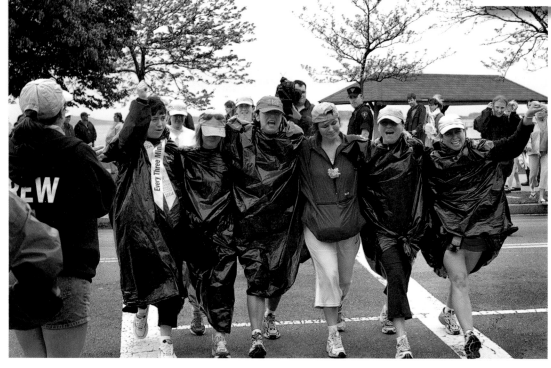

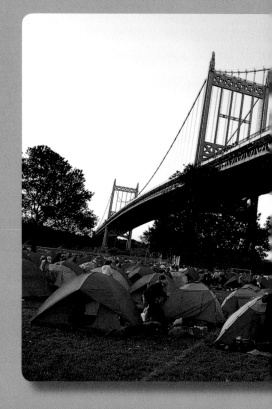

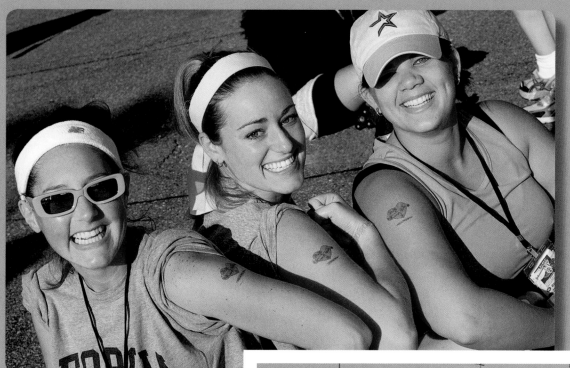

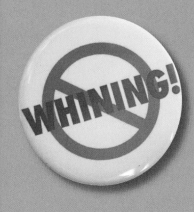

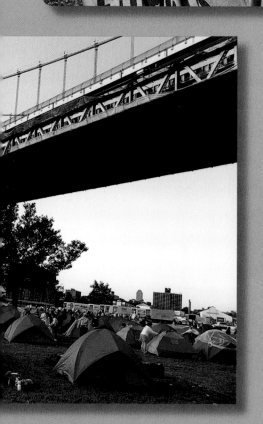

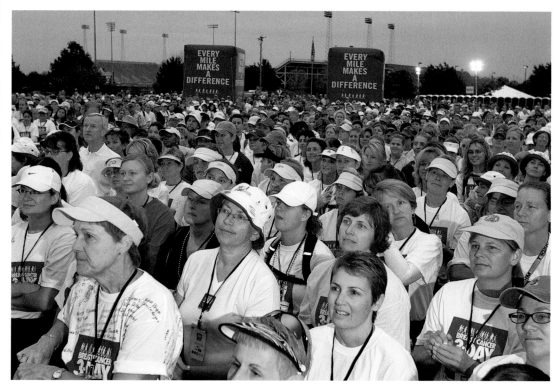

Rhonda Kirby

Kahnawake, Quebec, Canada

"Everyone is still talking about it, still on a high from the experience. All the girls are saying, 'We have to do it again.'"

Native American Rhonda Kirby literally brought all of her "Mohawk Spirit" to bear on the battle against breast cancer. Rhonda lives in Kahnawake, one of the seven communities of the Mohawk Nation. The name means "on the rapids," which is appropriate for this community of 7,000 residents on the banks of the St. Lawrence River a few miles south of Montreal.

Rhonda's mother was diagnosed with breast cancer in 1994, and although she successfully battled that disease, she later developed colon cancer and passed away in October of 2003. A couple of months afterward, Rhonda saw a magazine advertisement for the Avon Walk for Breast Cancer in New York. She knew immediately that she wanted to participate in the event. "I saw it as a personal journey to help with my healing," she says.

Rhonda soon found that she was not the only woman in her community who wanted to join in the battle against

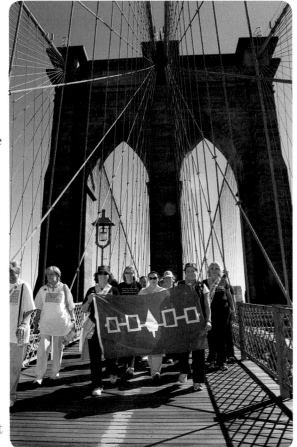

breast cancer. "I talked to a couple of close friends," she says, "and they said, 'Yeah, yeah, let's do it.'" Those friends talked to other friends, and by the time of the information meeting in Albany in April, the group had grown to about 12 women. Then they noticed on the event Web site that Team Avon had about 39 people on it. "We started thinking, gee, wouldn't it be something if we could beat Team Avon?"

More word-of-mouth networking swelled their ranks to almost 40, says Rhonda, and with "everybody really psyched up about participating," they began to dream of assembling "the biggest team ever." They invited the women from the neighboring Akwesasne community to join them, a strategy that basically doubled their numbers—and also necessitated a team name change from Kahnawake Spirit to Mohawk Spirit. When all was said and done, Rhonda was leading a

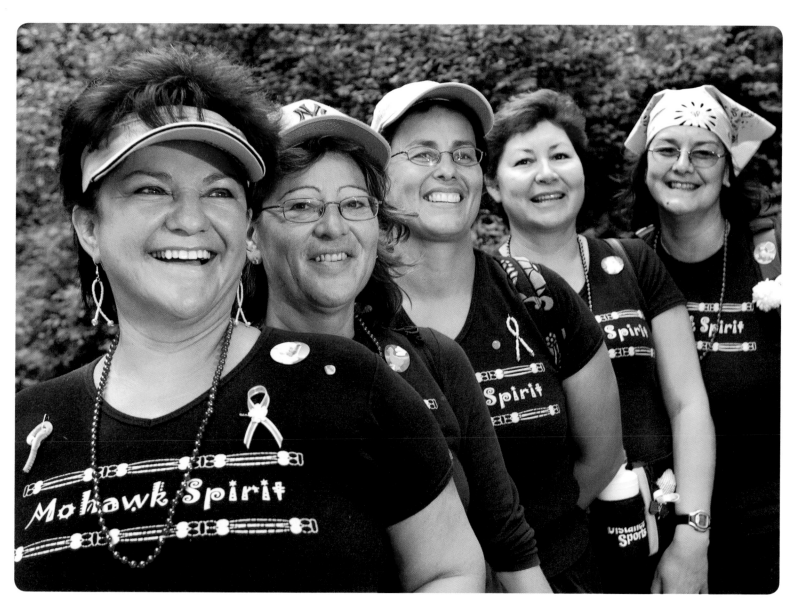

team of close to 80 women—including three survivors— into the New York event.

Needless to say, such a large number of participants called for some innovative fundraising. One woman re-

ported having heard about a "topless car wash" in Boston. It was advertised for two weeks, and on the day of the event, the TV and radio people were there, and cars were lined up for miles. The car washers were indeed topless—topless men. Rhonda's team replicated that brilliant ploy and netted $3,000 in one day.

Another idea they tweaked was Montreal's annual huge comedy fest, "Just for Laughs." Rhonda's event, "Just for Breasts," was a smashing "pink and black" affair, with the comedy talent from Montreal, a big auction, and bras hanging from the ceiling for decoration. That evening, says Rhonda, brought in about $8,000.

Add in receipts from sales of key chains and "Mohawk Spirit" bumper stickers, and by the time of the Avon Walk, the team had raised approximately $111,000 for the fight against breast cancer. "It was our first time," says Rhonda, "but we're real go-getters around here."

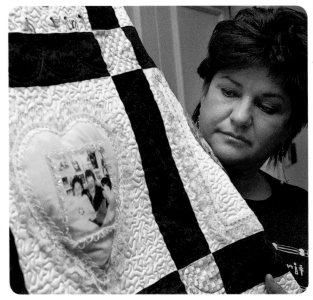

Mohawk Spirit also commemorated the event by collaborating on a beautiful quilt, for which one of Rhonda's close friends created a square depicting Rhonda's mother. "It is so beautiful," says Rhonda, "that it is really difficult for me to look at without crying." The quilt now hangs in a crafts shop in Kahnawake, says Rhonda, but the team is hoping that it will soon adorn a wall in the local hospital.

As for the walk itself, Rhonda describes it as "the experience of a lifetime." Crossing the finish line after walking 26 miles on Saturday was something she'll never forget. "We don't know whether we cried more or laughed more during the whole event," says Rhonda. "You know, at mile 21 it was getting pretty grueling. All you can do at that point is make sure you keep drinking water. And then you cross over that bridge and see everybody on the island waiting and cheering, and it's just like *Oh my God!*"

When Rhonda returned to walk across the Brooklyn Bridge for the closing ceremonies Sunday evening, "the tears were just pouring out. The whole thing—everyone still talks about it. We are still on a high from the whole experience."

Rhonda is delighted that her team raised so much money for such a worthy cause, and she also knows that all the local media exposure her team received had the effect of raising breast cancer awareness within the Kahnawake community. In fact, one woman has already told Rhonda that she went to get a mammogram after hearing about Mohawk Spirit, and, says Rhonda, "that makes all the difference in the world."

Perhaps best of all, though, is the immediate effect the experience is having on the women she participated with. Rhonda explains that part of her job is to promote healthy eating and daily exercise in her community as a means to combat diabetes, a prevalent problem among Native

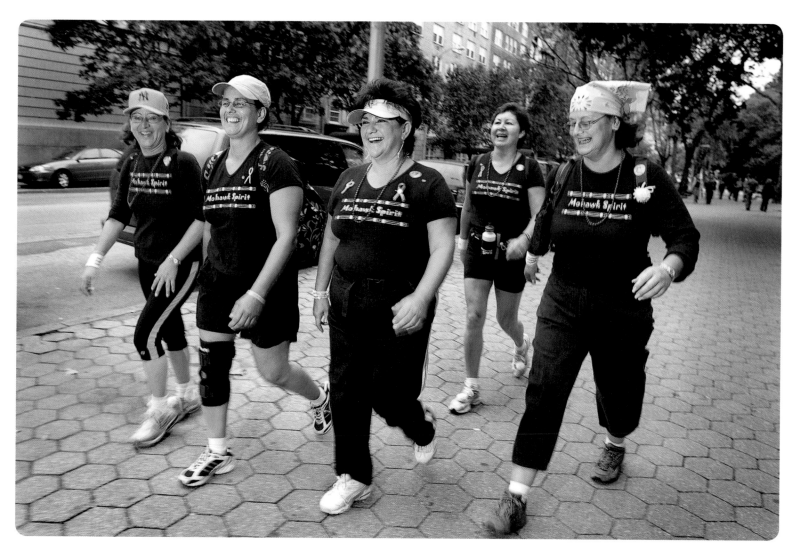

Americans. She realized that nothing could have suited that purpose better than preparing to participate in an Avon Walk for Breast Cancer. "I knew that if these women were willing to train for six months, they were not going to just stop walking after that event. So we have 37 women from Kahnawake who have made major lifestyle changes.

Their commitment to that change is evidenced by the fact that Rhonda is already making arrangements to lead Mohawk Spirit into the Big Apple again for the 2005 event. "We formed such a great bond," she says. "A lot of girls are saying they just can't see how it could stop."

Robin Steiner

Phoenix, Arizona

"I walk because I believe that if we don't get involved, we're never going to see an end to this disease."

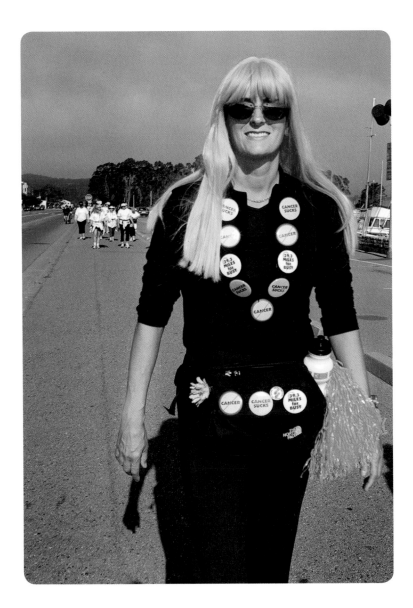

If you've been to an Avon Walk for Breast Cancer in the past five years, you've probably noticed Robin Steiner. In the first place, she's hard to miss, since her statuesque six-foot frame is topped off with a bright pink wig. In the second place, she has participated in practically every one of them. For Robin, walking in the vanguard of the battle against breast cancer has become a way of life—"a part of who I am."

It was 1999 when Robin first saw an announcement for an Avon Breast Cancer 3-Day. She was living in Los Angeles at the time, working in her successful floral design company and living with her husband, Wally, a Tiffany's executive. Robin had no personal connection to the disease, but she was intrigued. The Avon event was for a worthy cause, obviously, but what hooked her was the challenge of walking all the way from Santa Barbara to Malibu. She signed up, she says, "really just to see if I could physically walk 60 miles."

The event immediately became much more than a physical challenge. "Even during opening ceremonies," she recalls, "I was so moved by the people, by the strength that was in that crowd, by how everybody pulled together, by being in such a kind, caring environment, I just knew I was in the right place."

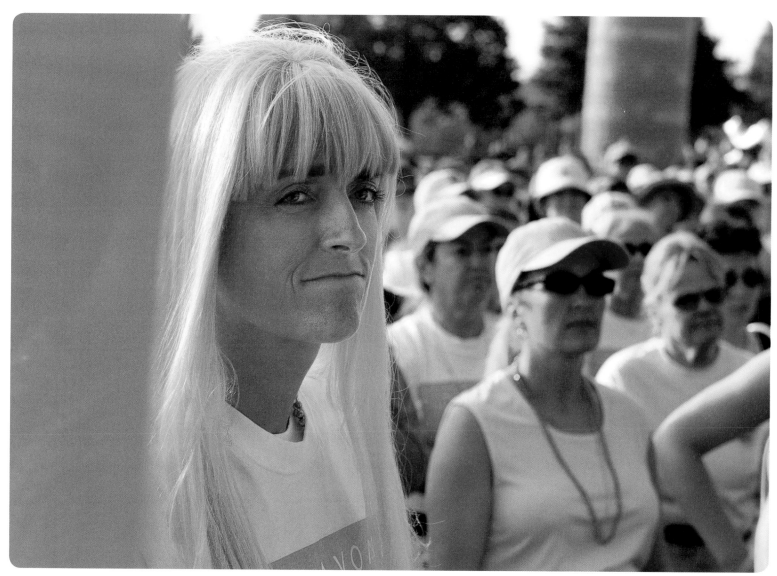

It was a place Robin quickly decided she wanted to spend more time in. She called home on the second night to tell her husband that Avon would be putting on seven such events in 2000 and that she planned to walk in every one of them. "Wally said, 'Yeah, we can talk about that

when you get home.' I said, 'We're going to talk about it a lot. I'm just warning you that I'm signing up now.'"

Robin had found her mission for her 40th birthday year. "I wanted to do something important, something real," she says, and walking 420 miles across seven different cities in

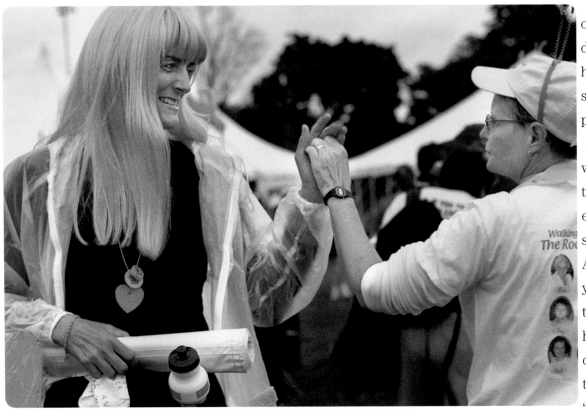

one of our friends had been diagnosed and had already had a mastectomy. All of a sudden, it started to get very personal."

At the end of 2000, Robin was officially the only person to have completed every event for an entire year. But she almost didn't make it. In Atlanta, the last event of the year, Robin hurt herself for the first time. She twisted her knee but kept going, overcompensating, and at the end of the second day "both knees were swollen,

the fight against breast cancer seemed a worthy ambition. Of course, she would have to raise the entry fee for each event, too, so her financial contribution would be significant. But walking for breast cancer is about much more than raising the money and logging the miles.

"All day long during the walks you're talking to survivors, or people whose mothers or sisters are on chemo, or people walking in remembrance," says Robin. "You're listening to these stories and you're growing close to these people. Then, when it was time to do Boston, I left on Wednesday, and by the time I got home Sunday night,

my ankles were swollen, and I was taped from thigh to ankle on both legs." She was in so much pain when she got up on Sunday morning, she knew there was no way she could finish the event, and she just broke down and cried.

She was still so upset standing in the breakfast line that a young woman she didn't know asked her what was wrong. Robin explained that her goal had been to do all seven walks, but that now she wouldn't be able to finish the last one. "I said, 'I can't believe it's the end of the year and I'll have to say I only did six and two-thirds.' This woman looked at me and said, 'You know what, honey?

Six months ago I finished chemo and I never thought I'd be here today, so you can do whatever you want to do.'" Robin says she wiped her tears away, went to the medical tent, and had them tape her up. "I walked every step," she says, "and I just made it, just in front of the sweep vehicle. I mean, I was one of the last four or five people in."

Robin completed her dream season, but she gives all the credit to that young woman. "She was a 34-year-old survivor, and I thought, *If she can deal with what she's going through, I can walk*."

In 2001, Robin decided to "cut back" and do only the "new" cities, cities that had not hosted an Avon event in 2000. She was on her way to one of those cities, Denver, when she saw a costume shop with pink wigs in the window. She couldn't resist. "I was planning to wear it just to the opening ceremonies," she says, "or maybe at the start of the

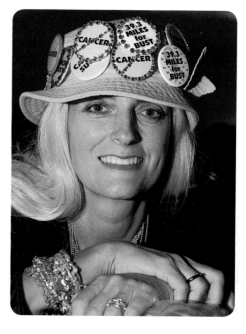

walk, then put it away. But people got such a kick out of 'the pink-haired lady' that I've been wearing it ever since. Now it's sort of my signature."

Trying to come up with new ways to fundraise, Robin has also become "the button lady." The hugely popular "CANCER SUCKS" button and the more recent "39.3 MILES FOR BUST" were both Robin's creations. In 2004, Robin says she came to New York with 1,000 buttons and returned home with 68, having netted $1,400.

By the way, in 2004 Robin was back to a full schedule, walking in all six Avon events. Her totals to date, in fact, are staggering: 23 walks, 1,200 miles, $88,000 contributed to the breast cancer crusade. "I feel like it's just part of me now," she explains. "It's what I'm supposed to do."

And if her pink hair and eye-catching buttons help recruit others to the cause, so much the better. "It just does good all the way around," says Robin. "It's good for people physically and emotionally, too. It's great just to have a reality check—to step back from your own little world and see how lucky you really are. It completely changed my life."

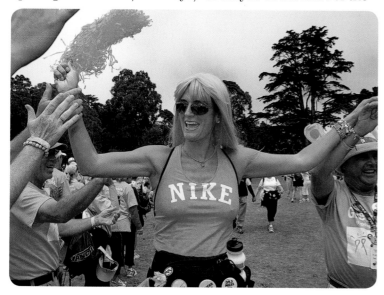

Trina Campbell & the Detroit Faith Walkers

Detroit, Michigan

"Our plan is to just not stop walking."

Girl, you're crazy." That was the response Trina Campbell got from her friends when she tried to put together a team to participate in the Breast Cancer 3-Day in Detroit. "I asked everybody I knew," says Trina, "and everybody I asked said no."

That wasn't the answer Trina was looking for, so she had "a little gathering" at her house. She invited about 20 people—colleagues, friends, family, husband—"everybody." She cooked them a big meal and then sat them down for a discussion. "I had done the research," says Trina, "and I told them everything I knew about it— the good parts, the bad parts, the money, the training, how difficult it would be. I just laid it all out there." By the end of the evening, Trina had seven recruits.

But the "discussion" wasn't quite over. Trina proceeded to inform the new team that she had already come

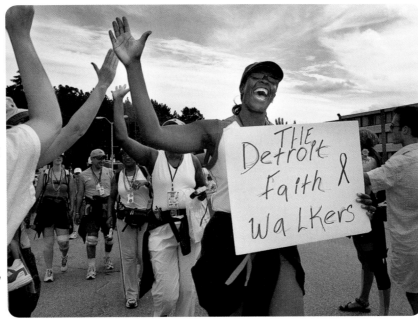

up with their name—the Detroit Faith Walkers. "They asked how I came up with that and I said, 'If we walk 60 miles, it's gonna be by faith.'" More generally, Trina explains that she really wanted a name with "a spiritual touch to it." Her first thought was simply "Faith Walkers," but, says Trina, "we added 'Detroit' to distinguish us."

As it happened, the group's membership evolved quite a bit after that first night. Some of the original eight dropped out, but as word of the group spread, others joined in. "People would see us on our training walks and start talking about us," says Trina, "and the word got around. Half of the team ended up being the result of word of mouth."

Trina says she was motivated to walk, in part, by the physical challenge of the event, but more important was the fact that her mother was a cancer victim. "It was lung

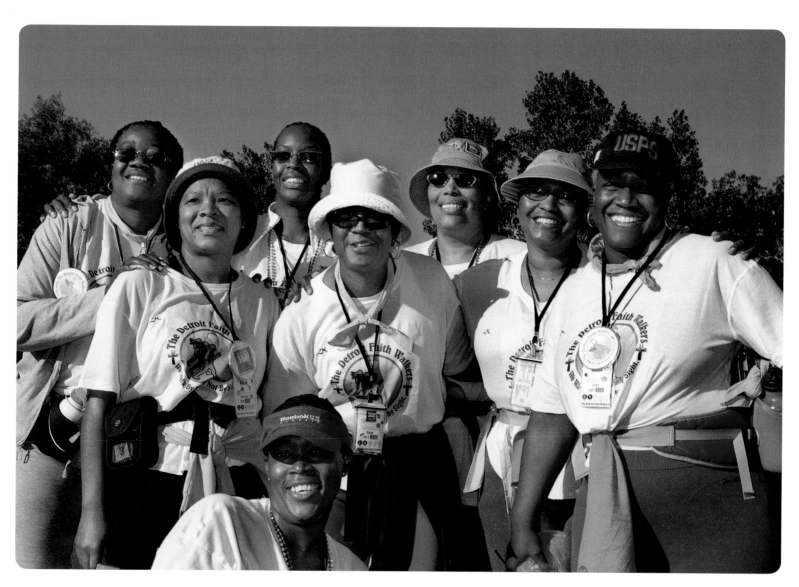

cancer, not breast cancer," says Trina, "but to me cancer is all the same demon. Cancer is cancer—no matter where it hits you." The Breast Cancer 3-Day gave her the chance to do what she had long wanted to do—walk in memory of her mother.

Other team members had their own reasons for participating. Debra Ann Smith says she walked "in memory of both my grandmothers who had breast cancer, and in honor of a friend who was diagnosed four years ago when in her early 40s." Charlotte Ankiel's mother is a 30-year survivor, and Charlotte also coordinated a stage 4 breast cancer research study, working with patients who in many cases did not survive. "I walk for all those people," says Charlotte, "so that one day they will be guaranteed a cure instead of just a hope for survival." Others, like Laurie Washington, simply wanted to give of themselves. "I walked because I am a woman," says Laurie, "because I am capable,

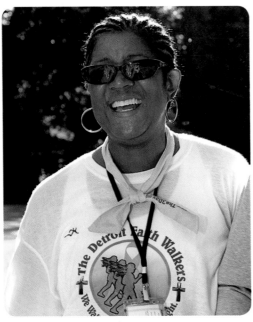

I care, and want to help make a difference."

Of the eight team members, Diane Walker was the single breast cancer survivor. She had been diagnosed in 1990, and for the last 10 years, ever since she passed "the 5-year mark," she had been intending "to do something to help others." She calls walking the 60 miles "the hardest thing I ever did in my life—and the most rewarding. It's just so worthwhile to accomplish something like that for a great cause."

As for Trina, her experience was so moving that she finds it difficult to put into words. The closing ceremony, especially, "was everything I thought it would be and then

some." But there was something about the whole event, including "the staff, the volunteers, everybody there just showing support," that Trina can only describe as "unexplainable." A big part of the magic was that "it was such a group of love. You just saw no hate anywhere. No color boundaries. No male/female, nothing like that. It was one big happy family."

Not that the walk itself was easy. "Motrin became our friend," says Trina, but everybody finished—including Diane Walker and Kim Edmondson, the last two people to come in to camp on Day Two. The reward for their perseverance was that they had the honor of hoisting the flag at closing ceremonies. "It was unbelievable," says Diane. "You come in last, and they treat you like you came in first." She says that after they raised the flag and sat down, "people we didn't even know wanted to give us food, water, they took off our shoes. They were like, 'What can we do for you?'"

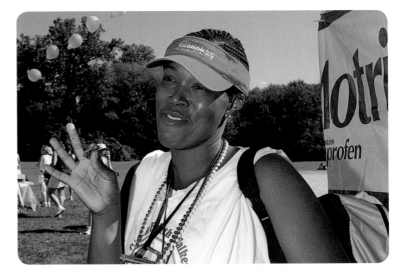

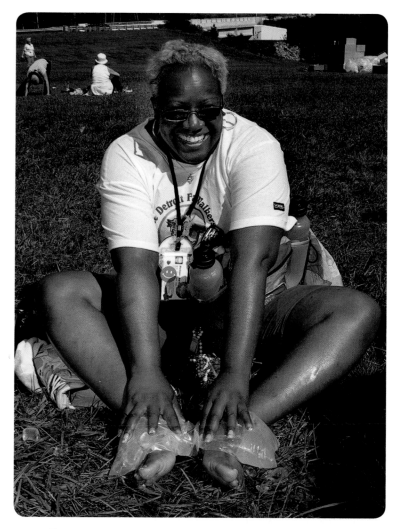

Detroit Faith Walkers will definitely be back next year—some as walkers and others as volunteers. Diane says she and some of the members have already decided to work one of the pit stops and are busy figuring out what their "catch" is going to be—maybe a Motown angle, she says.

But Trina says the team has discovered another important reason for staying together—to take the message of awareness into the black community. "We talked about that as a group," she says, "and that's one of the reasons we plan to continue." Raising awareness is now a team mission. "When you hear about the statistics and how high the incidence is for blacks, you really just say—well, wake up. Smell the coffee."

Accordingly, Trina says the team is working on ways to improve its visibility, including getting their name and specially designed logo registered and participating in a wider variety of wellness events. "To get our message out

"Diane and Kim refused to be swept," says Trina. "Their tenacity and determination were just great." Remembering "all the moaning and groaning" from the training walks six months earlier made Trina that much prouder when all her team members crossed the finish line. "Now we're still walking every Saturday morning at eight."

Having had such a tremendous experience, the

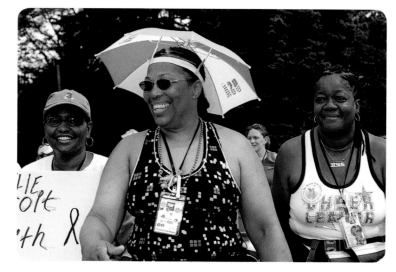

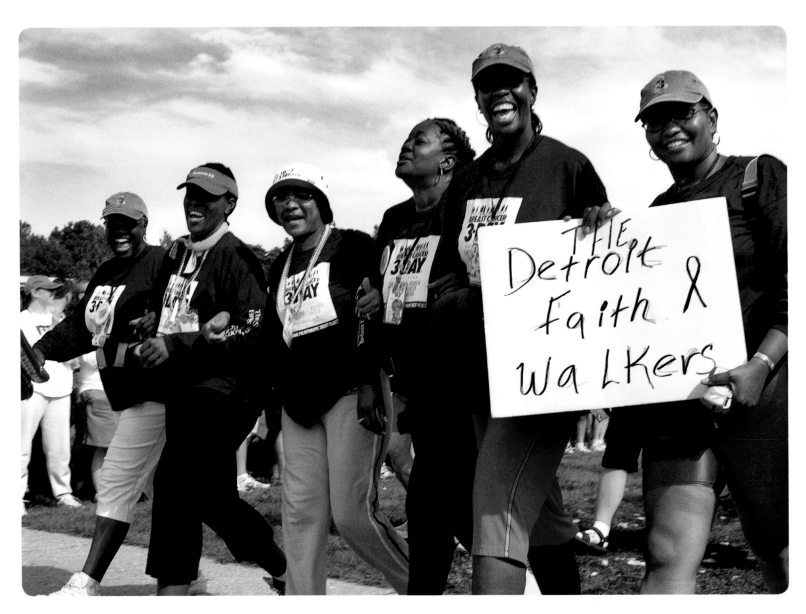

there, we want to get a lot more publicity," says Trina. "We want to really take this to a whole different level. We need to make sure that people are seeing us, that Detroit is seeing us. We want the community to know who we are,

what we stand for, and why we stand for these things. Our plan is to just not stop."

If the Detroit Faith Walkers needed yet another reason to continue their work, they got one via Trina's husband, a Detroit police sergeant. As Trina tells it, one of her husband's officers walked up to him shortly after the event and said, "I just want to tell you to tell your wife thank you." When her husband asked why, the man explained, "My wife has breast cancer and because of the money they raised, she was immediately able to have one of the surgeries she needed that our insurance didn't cover."

Nothing like instant gratification. "Here it is five days after the walk," says Trina, "and someone has already been helped by the money we raised. I was just so touched."

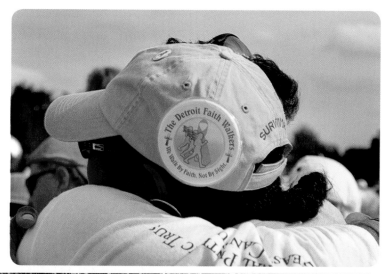

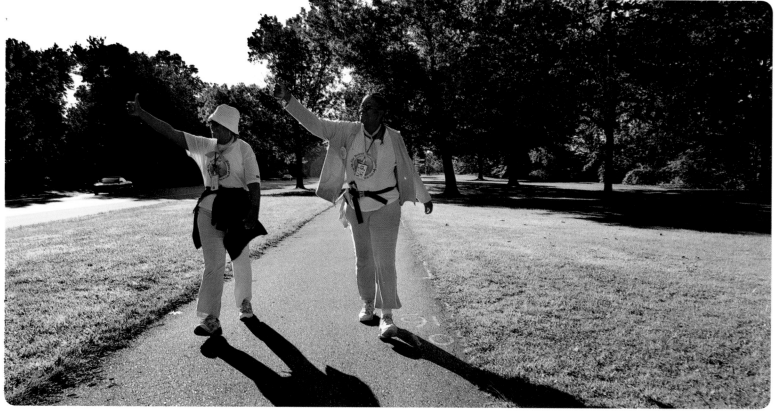

Barbara Jo Kirshbaum

Rancho Cucamonga, California

"I walk because I can't walk away."

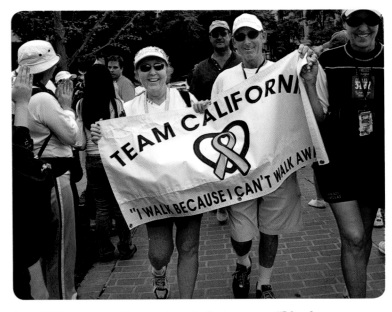

Barbara Jo Kirshbaum was 59 years old when she decided to participate in a 60-mile Avon Walk for Breast Cancer in 1998. A family counselor, she had several patients who were breast cancer survivors, and she well knew the importance of the cause. But, basically, she wanted to see if she could do it. "For me it was really all about the physical challenge."

She met the challenge in 1998, then again in 1999, 2000, and 2001. Along the way, she met Robin Steiner, who was walking every Avon event in 2000. She was impressed, she says, and a seed was planted in her mind. The seed germinated in 2001 when she ran into Nancy Mercurio. Barbara Jo had already planned to "go on a mission" in 2002 and had entered 7 events, but Nancy was signing up for all 13 Avon events that year and challenged Barbara Jo to join her.

The idea teased and tormented her. Could she do it? How much punishment could her now 62-year-old body take? "I kept talking about it and talking about it," she recalls, "but I couldn't commit. Just the logistics were overwhelming." When her husband, Bob, offered to handle all the logistics, deal with the travel agent, and find all the hotel rooms, Barbara Jo got on the computer and registered

for all 13 events. "Immediately," she says, "I had two emotions. First, I was proud of what I was setting out to do. Second, I literally wanted to throw up." Barbara Jo spent sleepless nights, filled with anxiety as she contemplated what she was asking of her body. "I don't take any of the physical demands lightly," she says. "I was a heavy kid and always the last one chosen for any athletic game."

But Barbara Jo did indeed participate in all 13 Avon events in 2002. Your calculator will confirm that that's a total of 780 miles—of *walking*. In the process she raised $90,000 for the Avon crusade.

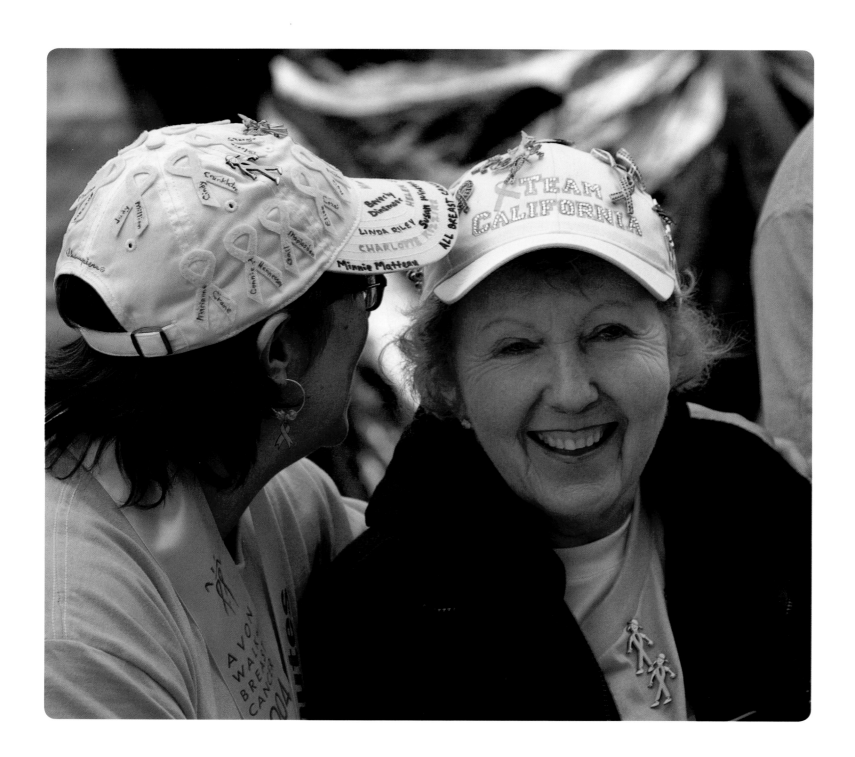

Was the petite grandmother now ready to collapse in her recliner and put those abused feet up? Not likely. Barbara Jo's quest was just beginning. It's like her sign says: she walks because she can't walk away. In 2003, she walked in all 8 events sponsored by Avon. In 2004, she walked in 5 of the 6 Avon Walk for Breast Cancer events and 9 of 10 Breast Cancer 3-Days. By walking those 804 miles, she raised $130,000 for the two organizations. The schedule for 2005? She'll walk 6 of the 8 Avon events and 10 of the 12 Breast Cancer 3-Days. "That's assuming everything holds up," she says, "like my body."

To date, Barbara Jo has walked in 42 breast cancer events and raised an astonishing $450,000. But she is quick to point out that the money comes not from her but from a host of wonderfully generous people. Like the guy whose company sprays her house every year, for example. Back in 1998, when she first realized that she would have to solicit donations from non-family members, he was one of the first people she contacted. It turned out that his

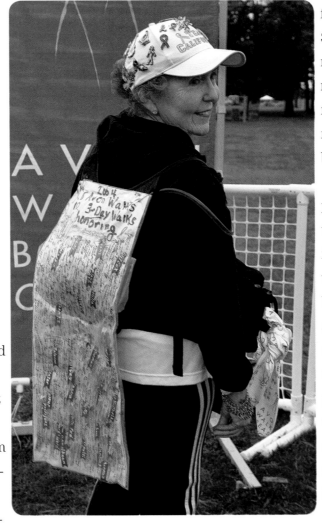

mother had recently died of cancer, and he immediately contributed $600, Barbara Jo's biggest donation that year. Within two years, his contribution had increased to $2,500; for the past two years it's been $5,000. "This is a guy I would not recognize on the street," Barbara Jo marvels. What she has learned from fundraising, she says, is that "you never know who has been touched by this disease."

At every event, Barbara Jo pays tribute to all of her contributors by wearing a capelike banner festooned with ribbons inscribed with their names. "I wear blue ribbons for my 'blue-ribbon angels' and white ribbons for all my other donors. Then, also, I wear pink ribbons with the names of all the people that my donors want me to walk in honor of. They really appreciate that, I think, and I'm sure I had more than 500 names on my banner by the end of this past year."

Barbara Jo is also eager to honor the achievement of her fellow walkers. When she is asked to speak at opening ceremonies, as she often is, she talks about the miles she has walked and the money she has raised "because that's what's on the script they give me." But she's not completely comfortable with that. "The last thing I want to do," she says, "is sound braggy or in any way diminish what these other great people have done. Anybody who raises $2,000 and walks 60 miles is a hero, and that's the message I try to reinforce."

The people to whom Barbara is most grateful are the members of her own family. They have all encouraged her enthusiastically, and all have walked beside her. Her son, David, walked three events in a row in 2004. Daughter Deborah walks when her teaching schedule allows. Daughter Ronda not only walks but also sells her beautiful "breast cancer awareness" jewelry, hand-fashioned from crystal and sterling silver, and

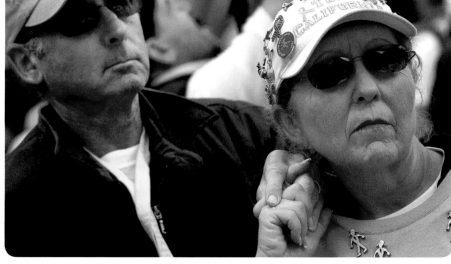

donates a significant percentage of her proceeds to the cause. Granddaughter Allison volunteered to have her hair cut off to participate in "Locks for Love." As Barbara Jo tells it, "When she was sitting in the beautician's chair, I told her she could still change her mind. She said, 'It'll grow back.'"

And then there's Bob. For the past two years he has accompanied Barbara Jo to every event. Originally his plan was to get her there and then, at the end of the day, make sure he had a nice hotel room to take her to for the night. During the day he would play golf. In fact, Bob has played no golf. Instead he spends all morning staying a few minutes ahead of the walkers, putting up signs (created by Ronda) that say things like "WALKERS KICK ASPHALT!" or "WHERE'S THE POTTY?" or "ARE WE THERE YET?" He puts up 30 or 40 signs per event, he says, or one sign every third to half mile along the route. Barbara Jo estimates he hung 1,665 signs in 2004. Says Bob, "You can't imagine the number of walkers who've come up and told me that, without those signs, they just wouldn't have made it."

For seven years Barbara Jo has been walking to raise money and raise awareness. Bob puts it more personally. "I've got five granddaughters, three daughters, and Barbara Jo. The work is not done yet."

Adrian Wilson

Sommerville, New Jersey

"I walk for my mom—and also for myself, because you don't know what may happen in the future."

Adrian Wilson was only 12 years old when her mother was diagnosed with breast cancer at age 35. Adrian didn't understand much of what was going on at the time, but she knew her mother had surgery to remove one breast one year, then had a second mastectomy the next year.

Twenty years later, in 2003, Adrian's mom tried to gather her five children to walk with her in a breast cancer event sponsored by Revlon. Adrian and her siblings were ready to go, but their mother died suddenly of a heart attack just before the event took place. When Adrian heard about the Avon Walk coming to New York in 2004, she knew it would be a way to fulfill her mother's wish and to ease her own grief at the same time. "It was good for me," she says. "I wish I could have done it before she died, but at least when I visited the grave site, I was able to tell her that I had done the Avon Walk for Breast Cancer. It made me very happy afterward. It was just a great thing to do."

Adrian herself, now 32, recently had her first mammogram, and it bothers her than not many women her age are encouraged to do the same. Her own gynecologist, even knowing her family history, told Adrian she was too young to worry about it, but the gynecologist was over-ruled by Adrian's family-care doctor. "She was the one who sent me to have it done," says Adrian. "She said, 'You are *not* too young. You need to go.'" In that sense, says Adrian, participating in the Avon Walk was something she wanted to do for her mother, for herself, and "for all young women who actually lost their mothers to cancer."

Adrian walked with her boyfriend, Dave McLaughlin, who didn't bat an eye at the prospect of the 39-mile trek. "When she told me she was walking in memory of her mom and asked if I would walk with her, I said, 'Sure.'" The fundraising didn't deter him either, says Dave. In fact, he hopes Adrian recruits him again so that he can "work harder and raise more."

The young couple trained together, too, but "not enough," says Dave. Adrian recalls that before the first day was over her feet began to tell her, "Okay, we're not going anymore—that's it," and Dave agrees that they were "definitely in pain." But you wouldn't have known it watching them stride across the finish line Sunday afternoon. "Hey," Dave explains, "our motive was the faster we walk, the sooner we'll get done."

Whatever her feet might have been saying, Adrian says, "Wonderful! Beautiful!" when describing the whole

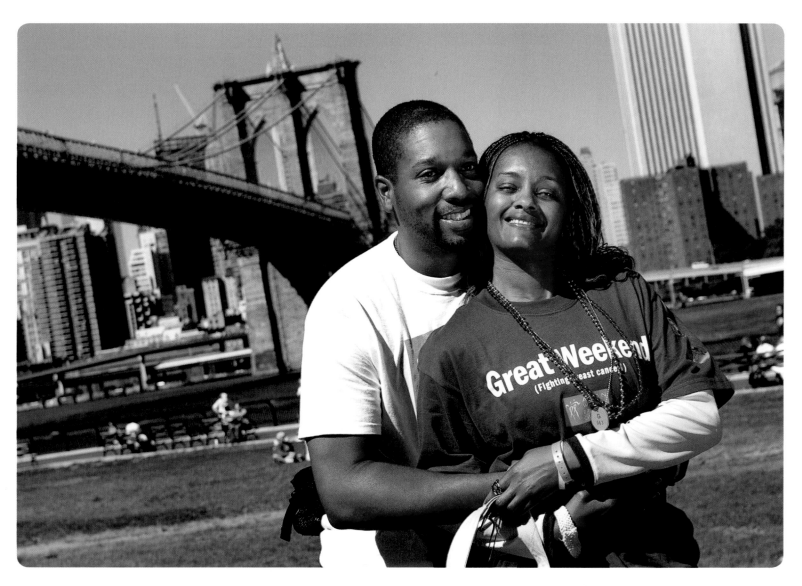

experience. "Meeting people from all the different parts of the country, hearing all their stories—it was just a great event." A special memory for Adrian was "a lady that was part of the cheerleading team." Adrian says she didn't know what the woman's motive was, whether she was a survivor or a victim's loved one or what—but it didn't matter. "As I walked by her, she was saying, 'Great job. Thank you so much for walking,' and I just really felt it emotionally. It felt like she had a deep appreciation for what we were doing and it was just so heartfelt—it really warmed me."

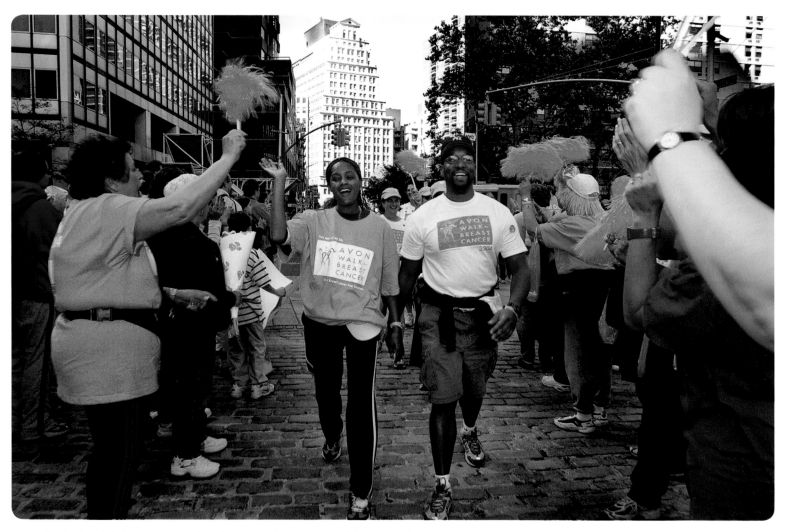

Still, for Adrian personally, the most important thing about the Avon Walk and other such events is that they get people talking—*communicating*—about breast cancer. Adrian says that in the case of her mother, only 20 years after the fact, when she was planning to participate in the Revlon event, did she begin to open up about her own experience. At the time she was diagnosed, says Adrian, "she was very secretive about it. You know, cancer wasn't a thing to talk about back in those days." It still pains Adrian that she never really knew what her mother went through. It pains her to think of her mother going through it basically alone. "I really wish I could have talked to my mom about it all," says Adrian, "but it was a hush-hush thing for a very long time."

All the better, then, that the walls of silence are coming down—which Adrian realized emphatically when she began fundraising for the event. "All these people were e-mailing me back saying, 'Yes, yes, I want to help because my mom had it.' Or people at work were telling me their aunt or grandmother had it. But I never knew it because for a lot of people it's still something they don't really talk about." Some of her friends, and even her sisters, cautioned her that it would be difficult to raise so much money, says Adrian, "but you'd be surprised how many people's lives have been touched."

What's more, when their friends and relatives realized she and Dave had completed the walk, "the stories really started pouring out," says Adrian. She found herself talking to the mother of a friend of Dave's, "who otherwise would have never said anything to me." Breast cancer—and what the Avon Foundation and other organizations are doing about it—is the subject of workplace conversations now, says Adrian. She has been asked by countless people what the walk was like, and she has encouraged them to "get out there and try it."

Closer to home, when Adrian got word that her uncle's wife had had a mastectomy and reconstruction surgery, she knew that she could call her up and talk about it. Not that such conversations are easy. "You don't really know what to say," Adrian admits, "but I called and we talked. We talked about my mom, and about her and how she was doing, and about her 10-year-old son, and how she

wants to be around to see him grow up." The exact words are not so important. What's important is that the door is open and that the silence and isolation are over.

Adrian realizes that her aunt represents the huge advance in the fight against breast cancer over the past 20 years—not only in that she could avail herself of a procedure not available to Adrian's mother, but also in that she felt free to talk about what she was going through. "That's why doing the walk and raising the money were so important," says Adrian. "I can see the difference it is making. Thanks to people like Avon, it is going to get better. It *is* getting better!"

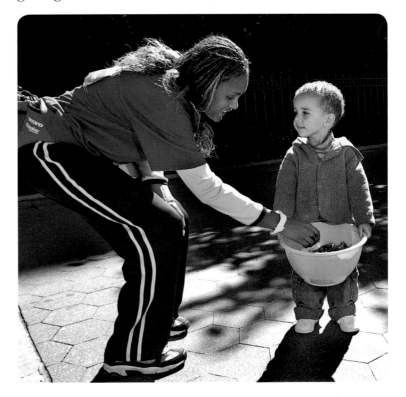

Lillian & Sue Williams

East Lansing, Michigan

"Everyone who attempts one of these walks is a superhero." —*Sue Williams*

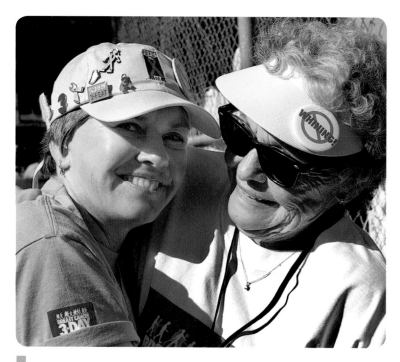

It's probably safe to say that Lillian Williams was the only 80-year-old walker in the 2004 Breast Cancer 3-Day in Detroit. Her daughter-in-law had been diagnosed with breast cancer in 2003, says Lillian, and she and her husband (Lillian's son) "were coping with it quite well" when Lillian's son suddenly died of a heart attack in December of that year.

With those sad circumstances in mind, her other daughter-in-law, Sue, a veteran of many breast cancer walks, approached Lillian with the idea of participating in the 3-Day. "I thought it was a good idea and wanted to do it," says Lillian, "after I got my doctor's okay."

She did wonder, though, how in the world she would be able to raise the money. "But Sue said, 'Mom, you're going to be surprised.'" Sue was right. Lillian sent letters to friends, family, and members of her two golf leagues, "and the response was fantastic." Says Sue, "Eighty percent of the people she sent letters to made contributions. She ended up raising $3,000."

A few weeks before the event, Lillian was in Denver visiting the daughter-in-law with breast cancer and happened to mention her big plan. Her granddaughter, Mary, "decided then and there that she had to do it, too," though, again, the fundraising was an obstacle, especially with only three weeks remaining. Lillian says she advised her granddaughter to "call Aunt Sue."

"I told her to get her ticket, get her shoes, and register," says Sue. About the fundraising, Sue felt confident that Mary would have the same kind of experience as Lillian, but reassured her that she would cover any shortfall. Not necessary. Mary raised over $3,600 in two weeks.

When Sue's daughter, Melissa, signed on and flew in from New York, the Detroit event featured three genera-

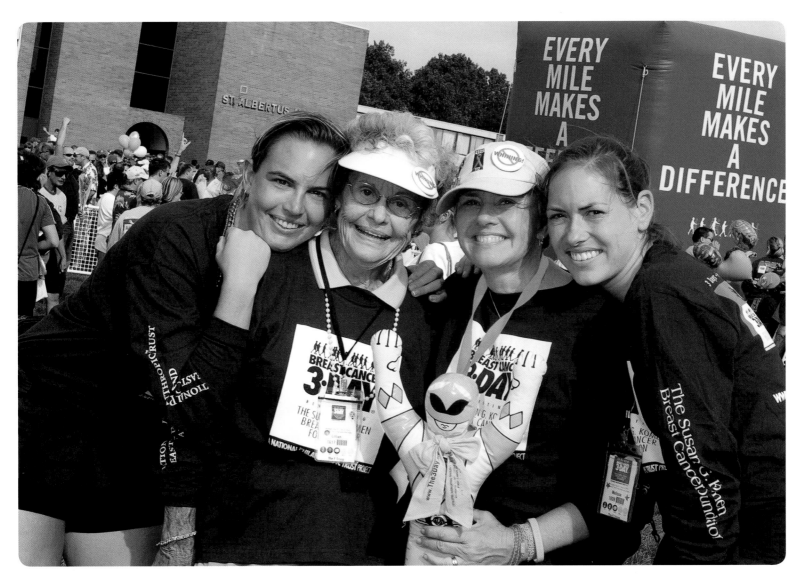

tions of the Williams family, representing a sizable portion of the continental United States.

There's no doubt about who the captain of this team is, though. The 3-Day in Detroit was Sue's fifth breast cancer walk, and it's hard to imagine a woman more dedicated to the cause. "I keep walking because I can," she says. Her commitment began several years ago when she lost a close friend to heart surgery and knew she needed to be in the company of "positive people." By the time of her third walk, for which she flew to San Francisco, both her sister and her sister-in-law had been diagnosed. "So now it has become very personal," says Sue. "Doing these walks is a way to help in the healing of my family."

But Sue is very much aware of the wider family as well. At the Detroit event, she pasted a sign on Lillian's

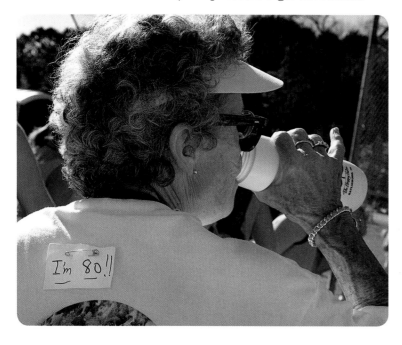

back saying, "I'M 80!" Melissa protested, and Lillian herself wasn't sure she wanted to make herself the center of attention. But Sue insisted that her mother-in-law's age was very much to the point. "I explained that the walk is all about inspiring others," says Sue. "It's about keeping others going and encouraging them to ask even more people to walk next year."

While Lillian walked with a sign on her back, Sue walked with a big Pink Power Ranger strapped onto her

own. It has personal significance. Her oldest daughter gave it to her during the closing ceremonies of Sue's first walk. "She said, 'Mom, you are my superhero,'" Sue recalls. Now, though, the Power Ranger is part of Sue's mission. "I wear it to make people laugh, to keep their spirits up, to encourage them. I feel my role now is to increase the numbers, to let people know that they will be inspired and empowered by doing this. So my message is that everyone who attempts one of these walks is a superhero. We are all doing something that most people wouldn't think about doing."

A lot of people don't think about doing it because the prospect of the 3-Day is so intimidating, as Sue realizes. Raising money, walking 60 miles—these are daunting tasks. "But when you hear that an 80-year-old woman participated, or that a woman signs up a couple of weeks before the event and raises the money without any problems, maybe you realize you can do it, too." The mistake, Sue says, is being afraid to try. "The biggest thing I tell people is not to let fear run your life. Step out of the box." After all, there's no downside. "Even if you don't make it, you've still experienced a lot more than if you'd never tried it."

And there's a huge upside. Sue points out that because of her mother-in-law's and niece's participation, another $7,000 was contributed to the cause. When you add in Sue's and her daughter's dollars, the total comes to more than $17,000. "That's starting to save lives," says Sue. In fact, Sue herself, over the past four years, has raised approximately $43,000. "But you'll never see my name publicized as one of the big donors," she says, "because on Day Zero, any money I have left over I give away to walkers who have come up short. That gives somebody else a chance who might not otherwise get one." Who gets the credit doesn't matter, says Sue. "The point is that my family and I know that the money we raise is making a difference."

As for Lillian, well, the Williams family is blessed with one game grandmother. "You need to understand that Mom never really got tired," says Sue. "She stopped after 15 miles the first day, but that was just because it started raining, and her hair was getting flat." Lillian stopped again after 15 miles on Day 2 to save energy for the final day, then walked another 10 miles on Sunday." She could have kept going, says Sue, but didn't want to get too tired to enjoy the end of the day.

"It was just fantastic," says Lillian. "I just loved the whole experience." And she didn't mind being "the celebrity" after all. She was touched and honored and

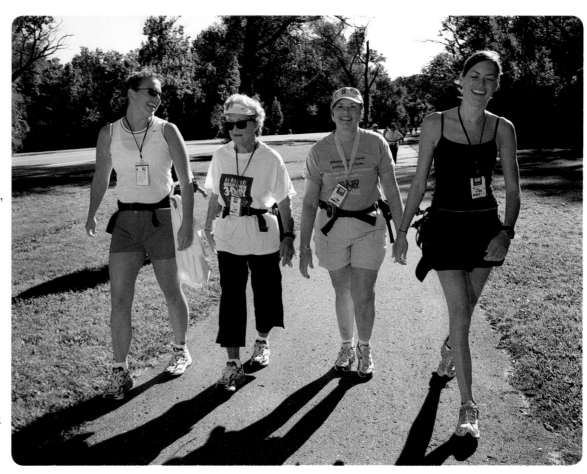

awestruck, she says, by all the younger women who wanted to have their picture taken with her. "I kept thinking, *Oh my gosh, here I am just an ordinary person, and I'm able to have the joy of doing something like this*."

Lillian says that when she first decided to participate, her friends were concerned. "They kept saying things like, 'Hope you'll be at the luncheon next week.'" But now, she says, "I've got the gals in my golf league all interested. It just goes on and on."

American Cancer Society
Making Strides Against Breast Cancer

Jones Beach—Long Island, New York

"When somebody comes up and tells you, 'Thank you for what you are doing,' you know your work is making a difference."
—Michele Chiulli

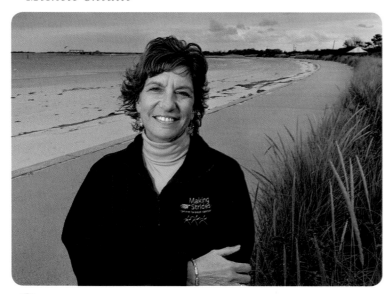

On October 17, 2004, in spite of a chilly wind and wintry temperatures, some 40,000 people poured out onto Long Island's Jones Beach to participate in the American Cancer Society's Making Strides Against Breast Cancer five-mile walk. Women, men, grandparents, babies in strollers—the entire community seemed to be there. Michele Chiulli, the Society's vice president for special events, Eastern Division, was especially moved to see a woman in a wheelchair with an oxygen tank, wearing her pink "SURVIVOR" T-shirt.

Michele remembers a time when things were different. She had been married for two years when, in 1971, her mother-in-law confided that she had found a lump in her breast and didn't know what to do. "I had no idea what to tell her," says Michele. "I had never really known anyone with breast cancer." Michele encouraged her to go to the doctor, but by then it was too late. "It was already in such an advanced stage. She lost her battle within eight months." Michele remembers how helpless her family felt, as if there were nothing anyone could do, as if they were the only people in the world going through such a terrible time.

In an odd and sad coincidence, when Michele married a second time in 1999, she learned that her second husband's mother, Edna Chiulli, had also died of breast cancer. This was in 1959, says Michele, "and they really had no idea then." So Michele says her career in the front lines of the breast cancer battle has personal overtones: "My work honors both those women—a mother-in-law, Lillian Schillberg, whom I loved dearly, and one I'm sure I would have loved but never got to meet."

The seeds of a new career were sown when Michele's first marriage took her from New York to Nebraska. "Being

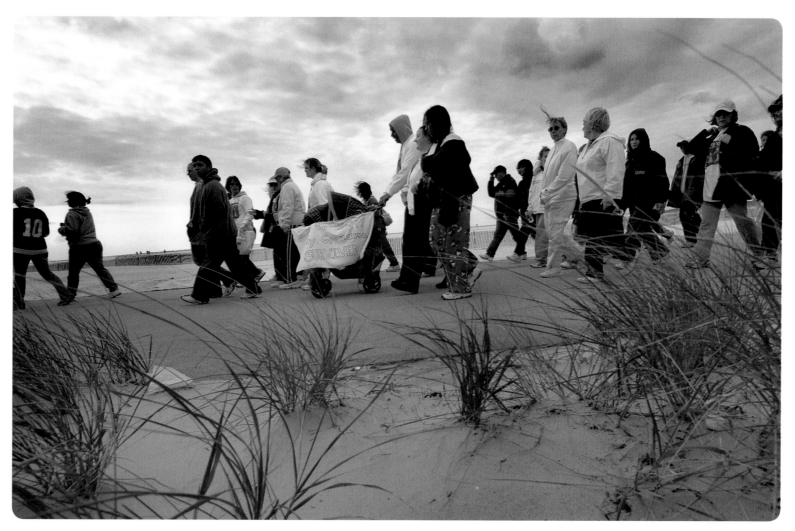

a Brooklyn girl, I started an arts organization there, and I found that I really loved working in the nonprofit arena." After moving back to New York, Michele spotted a want ad: the American Cancer Society needed a community organizer. She interviewed for the job and got it. "I think they hired me because they realized that if I could sell the arts to cowboys, I could sell anything."

That was 17 years ago. Because Making Strides Against Breast Cancer had its genesis in the Eastern Division, Michele was there at its inception. "We held the first fundraising event in New York state in 1993 at Rockwood Hall, Rockefeller's estate in Westchester," she recalls. "Three thousand people were there, and we raised $100,000, which, at the time, was truly amazing."

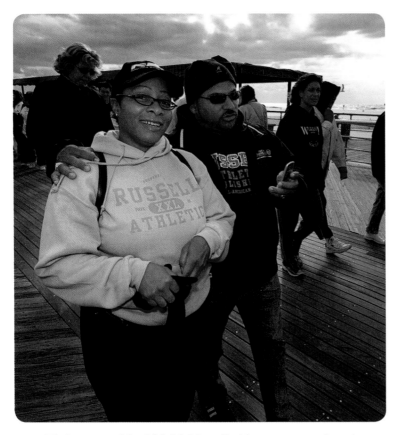

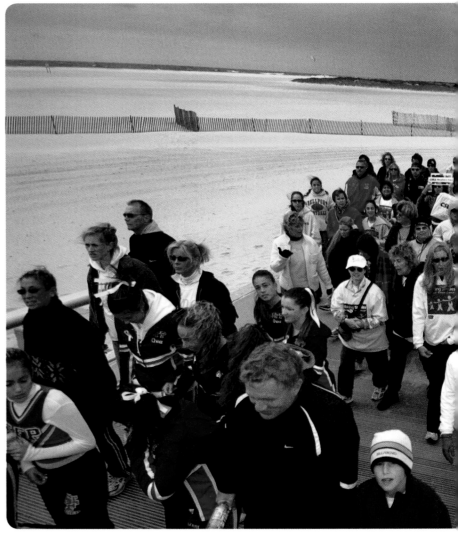

Today, roughly 100 Making Strides events take place around the country each year, usually in or near October, which is National Breast Cancer Awareness Month. Over the dozen years since 1993, Making Strides has raised approximately $100 million for the fight against breast cancer. For example, ACS researchers established the role of tamoxifen in the prevention and treatment of breast cancer, and the ACS also funded the research behind Herceptin, a monoclonal antibody that fights advanced breast cancer. "We really like to dedicate funding to new, innovative research opportunities," says

Michele, "which is one reason that 35 Society researchers have gone on to win Nobel Prizes."

That single event on Jones Beach raised $2 million, a sum as remarkable as the huge turnout. The size of the throng—as opposed to the relatively fewer thousands who participate in the long-distance cancer walks—is in part

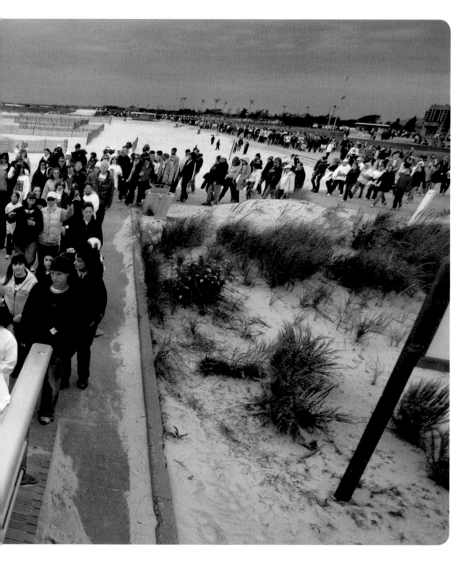

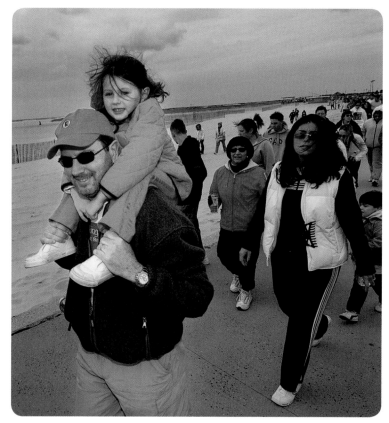

everyone is affected. And the more people we can reach, the more awareness is raised."

Michele also believes that the less stringent time and fundraising requirements help Making Strides events bring out the local community—which is the real target population. "We want to be reaching everyone, especially the women who are at work during the week. We want to bring the real demographics of the community to that walk." This is all the more important, says Michele, since those "real demographics" often also represent the underserved population of the community.

attributable to the fact that Making Strides is a five-mile event, so it offers the convenience of beginning and ending on the same day. Another unique feature is that no minimum fundraising amount is required for registration. In effect, then, Making Strides events are "open to everyone." This makes sense to Michele "because, directly or indirectly,

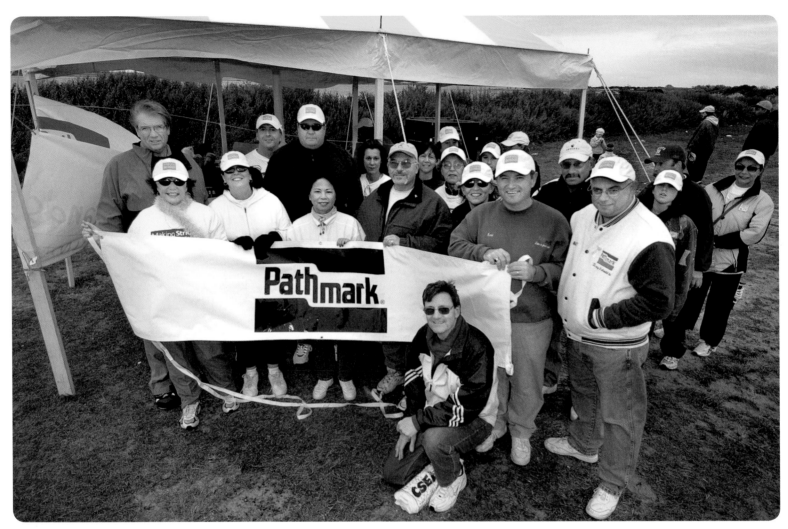

Much of the credit for Making Strides' success in bringing out the community goes to its volunteer program, which creates the necessary liaison between the local ACS office coordinating the event and potential walkers. "Basically, everybody tries to recruit as many team leaders as they can," says Michele, "and then those team leaders recruit the walkers." In 2004, in Eastern Division alone (New York and New Jersey), Making Strides had 10,000 team leaders, who in turn recruited 140,000 walkers. "Those volunteers are our infantry," says Michele. "They are our front line."

Even corporate sponsors get caught up in the "team spirit." Pathmark, for example, a multisite flagship sponsor at 15 sites for Making Strides, doesn't simply donate

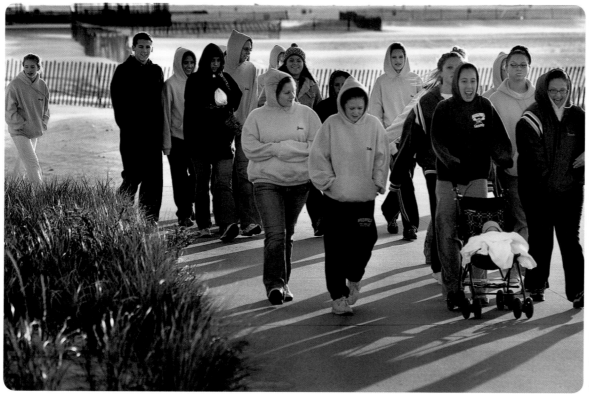

participants themselves—the breast cancer survivors and the larger community of family and friends who have been touched by the disease. The crowd at Jones Beach included Kimberly Russell, for example, who said she was there "because I'll be going through my second surgery tomorrow, and I am afraid to stop walking."

Likewise, Wendy Carley explained that six members of her family had had breast cancer and two had lost the

money and display its logo. As Director of Public Relations Rich Savner explains, "Every one of our 142 Pathmark stores has a team captain. Those captains recruit our own associates to walk, and we also invite customers to walk with us as part of our group at any given event." At sites like Central Park and Jones Beach, which Rich says are "big locations for us," you'll generally see 50 to 100 Pathmark people walking together. Such participation adds up. Rich estimates that since becoming a regional sponsor, Pathmark has raised more than $1 million for Making Strides.

Still, as with the long-distance events, the heart and soul of any Making Strides walk derive from the

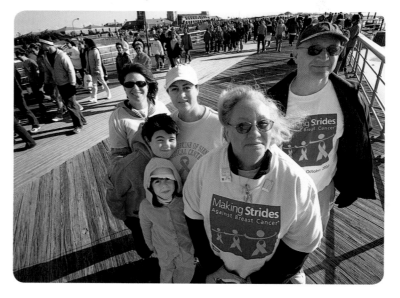

battle. "I will not allow this to happen to my daughter and granddaughters," declared Wendy. "We will win this fight!"

In fact, according to Jackie Wands, who as local ACS director of patient and family services has been involved with the Making Strides event on Jones Beach for eight years, the survivors' tent often provides the event's "most incredible experiences." In the first place, says Jackie, the tent is where survivors come to receive their special T-shirts, which in itself can be an overwhelming experience. "Just seeing that word *survivor* tangibly like that sometimes creates such sensitivity and emotion . . . there in that survivor tent is often where they just let it all out."

The survivor tent abets the work of another vital ACS program, "Reach for Recovery," which pairs trained breast cancer survivors with people just starting to deal with the disease. Often, says Jackie, breast cancer patients who have only talked to their "survivor partners" on the telephone have the chance to meet them in person at the survivor tent, and such meetings almost always overflow with healing emotion. In other cases, patients first discover this 36-year-old program when they are introduced to one of the survivor volunteers stationed in the tent. It's those volunteers, who donate not just their time but also their own stories of survival, that make the program such a success. "When they bring all that hope and experience to those patients and to their family members," says Jackie, "it is truly an inspiring thing."

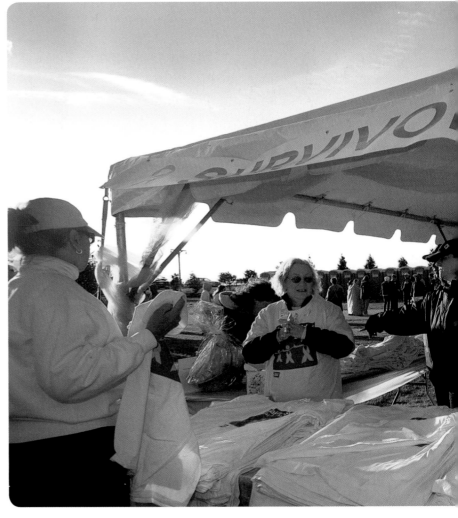

Money raised by Making Strides also helps fund the ACS patient program—"Look Good . . . Feel Better," an innovative service that helps women cope with the physical effects of their treatment. In a unique collaboration with the cosmetics industry, explains Jackie, patients are treated to a two-hour "makeover" and consultation with a professional cosmetologist. "The patients get great infor-

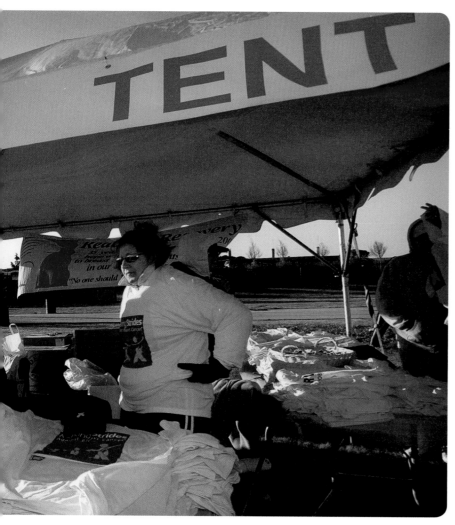

and an 800 telephone number that are up and running 24/7. "I really think this is so critical," says Michele. "If a cancer survivor or a caregiver is having a hard time—it doesn't matter whether it's three o' clock in the morning—you can call 1-800-ACS-2345 and talk to a live person. You will not get a recording. You can get some help any time, day or night." Michele learned the value of this service when a woman she had never met approached her to say "Thank you for what you are doing." She explained that she had called the 800 number and had gotten the help she desperately needed to get her sister through a late-night crisis. "That was kind of a defining moment," says Michele. "You wonder how many lives we touch that we're never really aware of."

With Making Strides Against Breast Cancer events across the country raising awareness, funding cutting-edge research, and providing innovative patient-outreach programs such as these, the American Cancer Society continues its historic mission: "Hope. Progress. Answers."

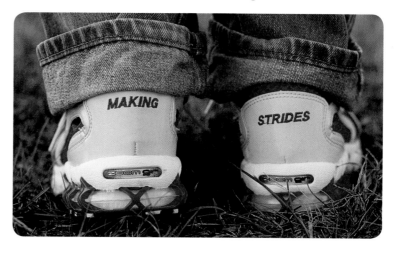

mation on skin care, advice on hair-loss issues like how to fashion a turban, and, thanks to the cosmetics companies, a cosmetic kit that's like a $250 value. It's the kind of thing that can really lift your spirits."

The fact that "cancer never sleeps" provides the rationale behind yet another ACS breast cancer initiative: the Society's "live information network," consisting of a Web site

Walking in
Memory

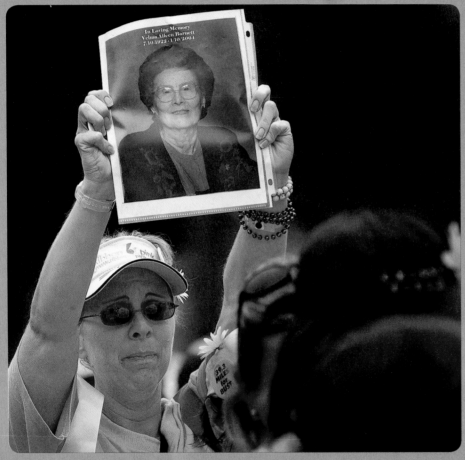

We also walk to honor all those lives lost to breast cancer. This disease doesn't care if you're short, tall, rich, poor, black, or white. It can strike any one of us, and it has left untold numbers of friends and family members with aching hearts—and deep memories. Often, during the special moments of our lives—weddings, bar mitzvahs, birthdays—those fond memories of the loved one who can no longer be with us give us the determination and courage to soldier on. And in walking to honor those lost, we find our own opportunity to grieve, to share, and to heal.

I walk because...

"It's something positive that I can do with my pain. I lost my best friend to breast cancer six years ago. The love of her friends and the best that medical science had to offer could not save her. If the money that I raise can keep someone else from dying, then my grief is somehow redeemed." —*Kathy Ellis*

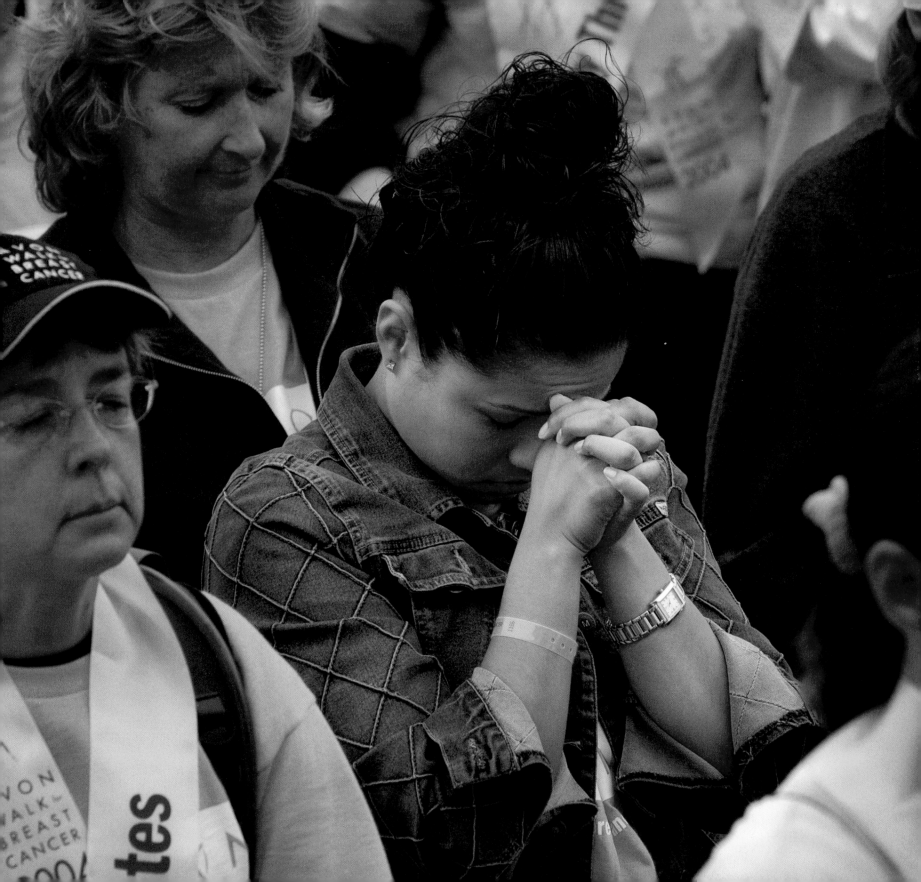

Ray Amaral & Wendy Simeone

Plymouth, Massachusetts

"I realized I was walking for all people who had breast cancer or who will have breast cancer, and the pain you feel in those final miles is very much a part of that revelation." —Wendy Simeone

For two and a half years Daria Amaral battled breast cancer. For two and a half years, her husband, Ray, and her best friend, Wendy Simeone, fought by her side. "She told me the day she was diagnosed," says Wendy. "We were standing in the parking lot outside the school building, and she told me she had breast cancer."

In 2003, Daria had finished chemotherapy and her cancer seemed to be in remission. She and Ray, after having been together for almost seven years, got married in October of that year. "It had been a good year," says Ray. "She had been doing pretty well. We thought maybe it was done." But Daria's cancer was aggressive.

"The picture kept getting more and more bleak," says Wendy. "Every time she turned around it was more bad news." The first terrible blow had come early on, when she awoke from her initial lumpectomy and the surgeon told her that the lump was much larger than she had anticipated—close to the point of being inoperable. "Then of course the next piece of news was that the cancer was out of the breast. That meant lung cancer and then eventually brain cancer, and then it was in her left hip . . ."

Ray and Daria's house was filling to the rafters with angels and candles—gifts of hope from friends and family. Eventually, says Wendy, Daria told Pam Borgeson, another close friend, "I'd rather have someone walk. Walk the Avon Walk and give money to fight against breast cancer."

Wendy and Pam agreed that if that's what Daria wanted, they would walk. The problem was that the Avon Walk in Boston was only five weeks away, leaving very little time to raise the $1,800 apiece. "We decided we would go anyway," says Wendy. "We would just write the checks ourselves."

They didn't have to. In five weeks the two friends raised more than $9,000. "The way the community came out to support Daria was overwhelming." Daria, an arts teacher, and Wendy, an English teacher, had been among the original faculty when their high school in the Plymouth Carver district opened in 1986. "Daria was the high school's only arts teacher, and she was absolutely beloved. When the superintendent told us we could fundraise at the school, the support was just incredible." Students sold pins "like crazy," says Wendy. The teachers purchased days to wear jeans. Everybody wanted to help. Then Wendy e-mailed a solicitation to her husband and asked

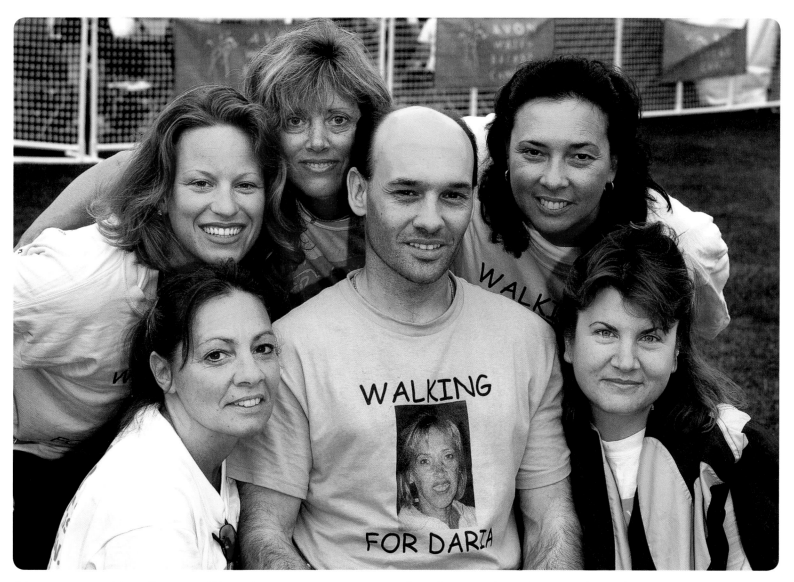

him to contact his colleagues. "Complete strangers were going online and giving us money," she says.

With enough money raised, five women now wanted to walk for Daria, including two of Ray's sisters. Ray wanted to join them, but Daria dissuaded him. He had had a hernia operation a few months earlier, but that wasn't the problem. "Daria had taken care of me. I felt fine. She just didn't want me to go." Wendy helped talk him out of it. "I told him Daria needed him," says Wendy. "The thing was, she didn't want him out of her sight."

Ray, says Wendy, was the love of Daria's life, and he never gave up hope. "I always thought she would make it," says Ray. "We were still fighting," adds Wendy, "as long as Daria was fighting."

On May 12, three days before the Avon Walk was to begin, Daria's long struggle came to an end. Family and friends held their wake the very night before the walk. During the evening, Ray told Wendy, "Well, I can walk now. I can't save her. I can't bring her back, but I can walk. It's the only thing I can do."

He hadn't trained, and he showed up in hiking boots, but he walked 39 miles for Daria. "My feet were fine," he says. "I never thought about them. It was like some driving force was pushing me the whole way, and then, once it was over with . . ."

Wendy remembers walking side by side with Ray during the final miles of the marathon. "I cried a lot over those last three miles," recalls Wendy. "Only then were all the implications of the act becoming clear to me. I had been so busy as a caretaker, both for my father [who had died just days earlier] and for Daria. There had been no time for contemplation, or for acceptance. We had all just been scrambling around madly."

But in those last three miles, says Wendy, the reason for the walk—the real meaning of the walk—became clear. "Yes, I was walking because Daria wanted her friends to walk. That was the motivation. But I discovered I was walking for a lot more than that. I was walking for all the people who had breast cancer or who will have breast cancer, and the pain you feel in those final miles is very much a part of that revelation."

In Wendy's case, walking for breast cancer hadn't been a choice she had made, hadn't been something she weighed in her mind or thought about the significance of. She had walked because her dearest friend had asked her to. But as one long mile led to another, a deep insight emerged. "Only in those last miles," she says, "did I see that what I was going through mimicked the process of suffering that I knew so well from having gone through it with Daria. I know it seems like a callous comparison, but when there are 5 miles left, it feels like there are 10 miles left. You are in agony; it is a process of constant letdowns. You want it to be over, but it is a long way from over."

Wendy remembers whining to herself as she looked around the harbor; the distance still to go seemed impossible, and demoralizing. "I felt just so let down," she says. "My husband said later, 'Why do they have to do it like that—with the 26-mile walk and the 13-mile walk? Isn't just raising money the whole idea?' It wasn't until those last few miles that I understood why they make it so grueling. It's because Daria, and so many others, fought so hard to stay alive."

Once they crossed the finish line, Wendy and Ray staggered to a nearby fence rail and sat down and cried. "I never really got emotional until we crossed the finish line," says Ray. "Then it all came out."

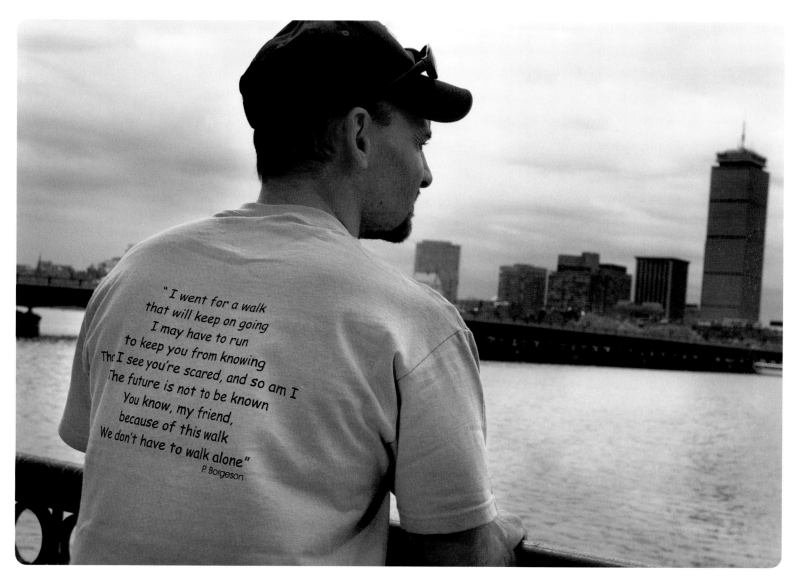

"I went for a walk
that will keep on going
I may have to run
to keep you from knowing
That I see you're scared, and so am I
The future is not to be known
You know, my friend,
because of this walk
We don't have to walk alone"
P. Borgeson

They consoled each other in the knowledge that it was good to have done this. Daria had wanted them to, and their promise to walk had made her happy. "It was the only thing we felt we could do," says Wendy, "that might make a difference—if not for Daria maybe for somebody else."

Wendy and Ray realized something else in that last stretch: that in spite of the pain—or rather because of the pain—they would be back next year. "Nobody is going to talk me out of it," says Ray. "I'm definitely walking again."

"Yes," agrees Wendy, "something happened on that walk."

Nancy Mercurio

Spokesperson, National Philanthropic Trust Breast Cancer 3-Day

"Everybody wants my job. I mean, everybody wants my job."

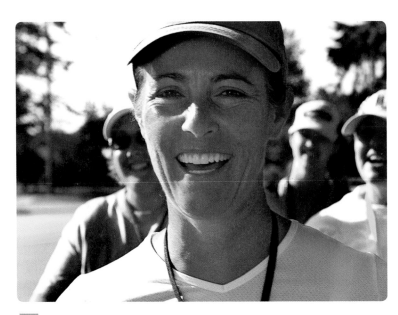

Funny how a little shopping at Nordstrom's can change a life. That's what Nancy Mercurio was doing when she saw a flyer announcing a Breast Cancer 3-Day Walk sponsored by the Avon Breast Cancer Crusade.

The announcement caught her eye because her mother, Oneta Deleo, had died of breast cancer less than two years earlier. Nancy, the only daughter, had been especially close to her mother, whose "incredibly positive outlook" kept her going strong for 11 years after her diagnosis. In 2000, the year after Oneta's death, Nancy ran the Paris Marathon in her mother's memory.

It was the following year, 2001, when she saw the display in Nordstrom's. "I thought, *I'm athletic. I could do this, and I want to do this for my mom,*" Nancy recalls, and sure enough, she could. She walked the Avon 3-Day Walk in Los Angeles in October 2001.

"It was the best thing I have ever done in my life," says Nancy. "At the opening ceremonies, I just cried my heart out. I must've needed to do it." Once the walk began, Nancy was walking by herself but hadn't gone too far before she saw a particularly rambunctious team "with these pink things in their hair." It was Barbara Jo Kirshbaum's team, Nancy recalls, and immediately Barbara Jo's daughter asked Nancy to join them. Nancy was so overwhelmed by the experience of the first day—meeting so many wonderful people, doing something that really made a difference—that in camp that night she signed up for another one. In camp the second night, after another incredible day of sharing commitment, she signed up for yet another. But then she met Roberta de la Santos, who had walked every single event in 2001, and with Roberta's inspiration, Nancy signed up for two more before the event was over.

Well, if you're going to do four . . . When Nancy saw Roberta again a few days later, she confessed to her real

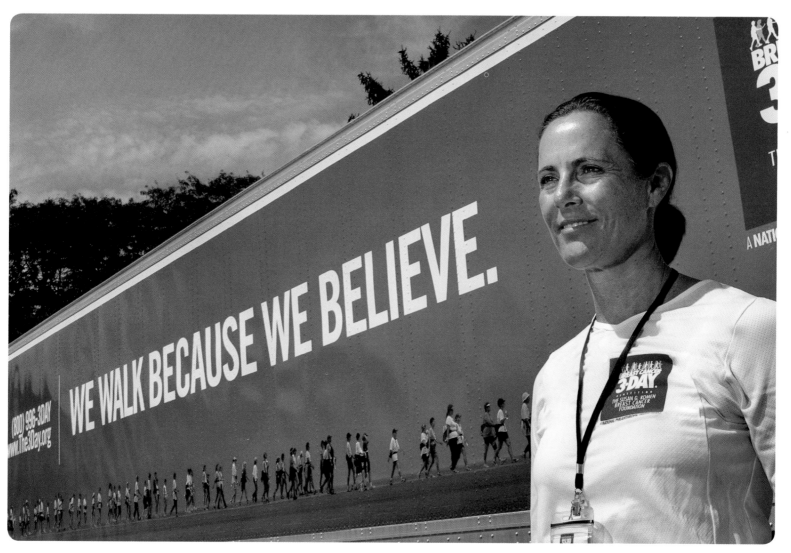

ambition. She wanted to walk every Avon event in the coming year. Roberta cautioned her that there were going to be 13 3-Day events in 2002, and when Nancy balked, Roberta told her that 18 were scheduled for 2003. That settled it, Nancy recalls. "If I'm going to do this, I need to go ahead and do it now." Shortly thereafter, she got an e-mail from

Barbara Jo Kirshbaum saying that she had signed up for seven 2002 events. Nancy e-mailed back to say, "Hey, I have to tell you something. I just signed up for all 13."

Given that each event demands walking 60 miles, 13 events would seem pretty daunting. But Nancy says the physical challenge didn't faze her at all because "one,

I don't get blisters, and, two, I have my dad's legs." But the actual walking is only part of the challenge. To participate in an event, you've also got to raise $2,000. Nancy hadn't worried about it; she had raised $18,000 for the Paris Marathon. But as the first event approached, she says, "I hit a brick wall." She was getting nowhere. She was glad she hadn't told many people about her plan to walk all 13 events because now it looked like she would be backing out of at least some of them.

But then it came to her: at three a.m. on a Sunday she sat up in bed with two words on her lips: "GOT MAMMOGRAM?" The first thing she did that morning was run a search to see if the phrase was copyrighted. It wasn't. Then she took the $5,000 bonus she had just received at work and headed for the local T-shirt company, where she purchased $5,000 worth of shirts, hats, and pins—all emblazoned with her new catchphrase. From then on, her practice was to show up at an event with a duffel bag full of her merchandise and sit down with a sign that read: "WALKING IN ALL 13 IN MEMORY OF MY MOM." "People were incredibly generous," says Nancy. "They would say, 'Here's $40, keep the change.' One woman wrote a $250 check for a $20 T-shirt."

That was the end of Nancy's fundraising difficulties, and she completed her "dream season" of walking in every 3-Day—780 miles in memory of her mother. But her work for the battle against breast cancer was just beginning.

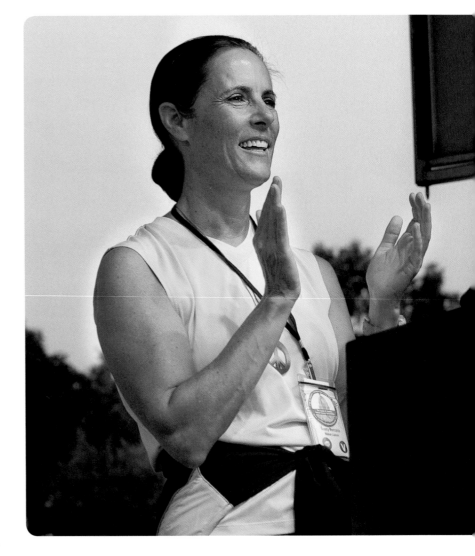

During the course of that 2002 season, by sheer serendipity, media-shy Nancy became not just a walker and a fundraiser but a speaker as well. It began casually, when she consented to a couple of interviews in the local media. But her story was compelling, and she obviously spoke from the heart. By the end of the year, she was a featured

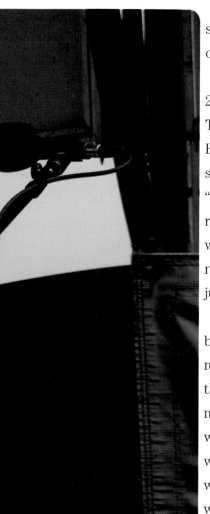

speaker at both the opening and closing ceremonies of every event.

An even bigger opportunity arose in 2003 when the National Philanthropic Trust teamed with the Susan G. Komen Breast Cancer Foundation to create a series of three-day breast cancer walks. "NPT knew they needed somebody to represent the walkers, to bring in the walkers' perspective," says Nancy. They needed a "spokesperson," and Nancy just happened to be in the job market.

In fact, the timing couldn't have been more fortuitous. Nancy had been making a very comfortable living as the chief financial officer for a small medical device company. But work was one thing, and the "incredible world" of the Breast Cancer 3-Days was another. She had returned to work after one event and overheard her boss complaining about her absences—despite the fact that "he was not inconvenienced one bit." "How many more of these things do you have to do?" he asked her. "I went out at lunch, got a home equity line of credit for $50,000, then walked back in and quit."

Quitting one job without another in hand was "probably the most irresponsible thing I've ever done," says Nancy, and the sudden career change has necessitated a serious lifestyle adjustment. She sold her house in San Diego and began renting a smaller place near the beach, but even that was too expensive. With that lease almost up, Nancy's next move would be into a two-bedroom apartment that would cut her rent substantially. She is "scaling way back," she says, "and it's taken a while to ease into that."

Her paycheck may be smaller now, but Nancy doesn't lack for compensation. "Here's an amazing thing," she says, "These people come out here and walk 60 miles, they raise $2,000, and when it's over, they come up to me and say, 'Thank you.' Isn't that phenomenal?"

Clearly, working for a great cause brings immense satisfaction. As Nancy puts it, "Everybody wants my job. I mean, *everybody* wants my job."

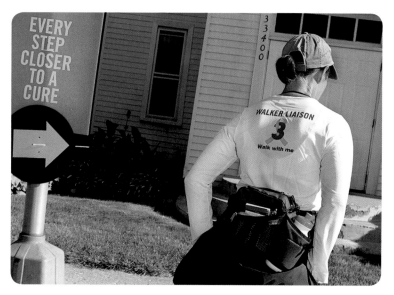

Remembrance

"Wearing our hearts on our sleeves—literally." You'll see many walkers wear or carry items while they walk in tribute to a family member or friend who has died from breast cancer. It's a way of saying, "This is why I walk." Sharing stories—some happy, some sad, some outrageously funny—with other walkers on this journey helps us remember that we are not alone. And although we may be walking for different people, we are walking for one cause: to find a cure.

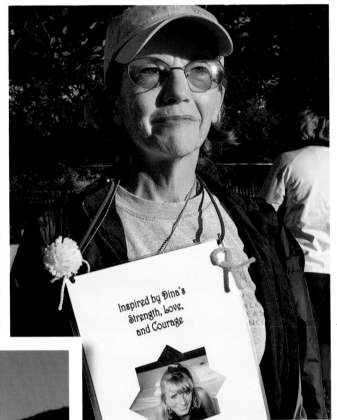

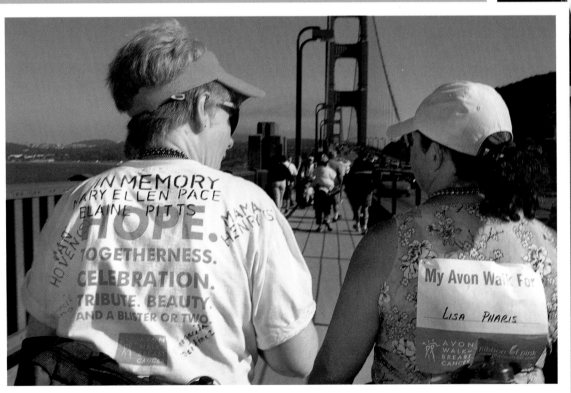

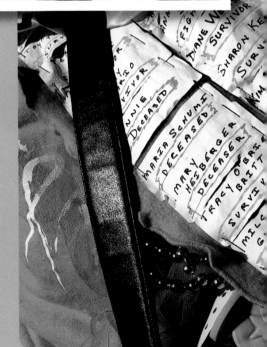

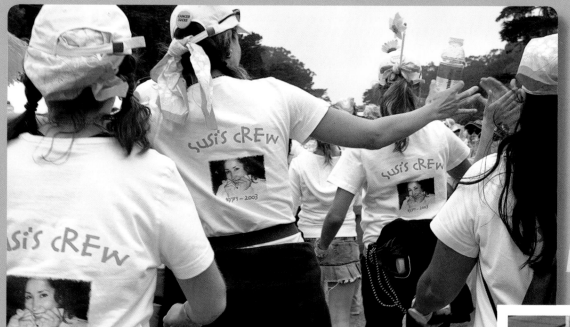

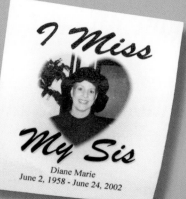

I Miss
My Sis

Diane Marie
June 2, 1958 - June 24, 2002

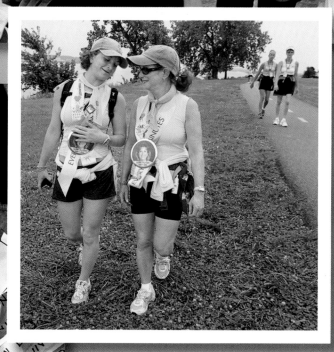

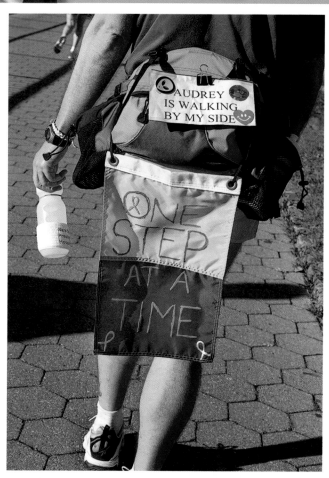

AUDREY IS WALKING BY MY SIDE

Mike McElduff & Peggy's Spirit

Fishkill, New York

"The cure will be found. I know it's going to happen, and I'm going to be there to see it—God willing."

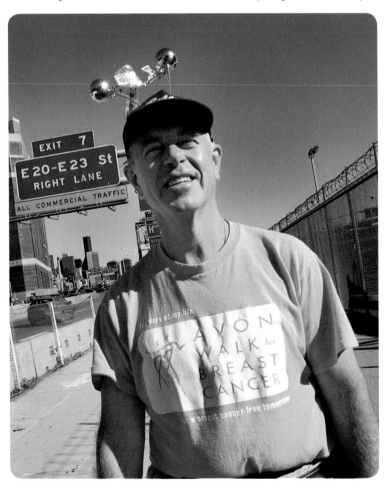

Peggy McElduff was born in 1925, the youngest of 10 siblings. Her daughter Kathleen Lyons describes her as "always full of life—a wonderful aunt, a special friend, a loving wife, a giving sister, a devoted grandmother and an incredible mom to 11 children." Peggy was diagnosed with breast cancer in 1968 and survived for 11 years, "which allowed her time to be with all those she loved and leave a little piece of herself for us to cherish and share in our everyday lives."

No wonder, then, that though Peggy died in 1979, "Peggy's Spirit" is very much alive. It is embodied in a team of her children, their cousins, and close friends who have devoted untold hours and many thousands of dollars to the fight against breast cancer, a fight they say they will continue until a cure is found.

The team had its genesis in 2000, when daughter Maggie McCann visited the "tent city" at an Avon Breast Cancer 3-Day and was filled with excitement by the event. The idea took wings the next year when Maggie and two of her sisters, Kathleen (Lyons) and Tricia Rothberg, participated as "Peggy's Spirit" in the Avon Walk in New York. Their older brother, Mike McElduff, the firstborn of Peggy's 11 children, volunteered at the event, giving tent assignments to the walkers. He was hooked.

"I just loved the people," says Mike. "They were so vibrant, so excited. Some were pregnant, some were

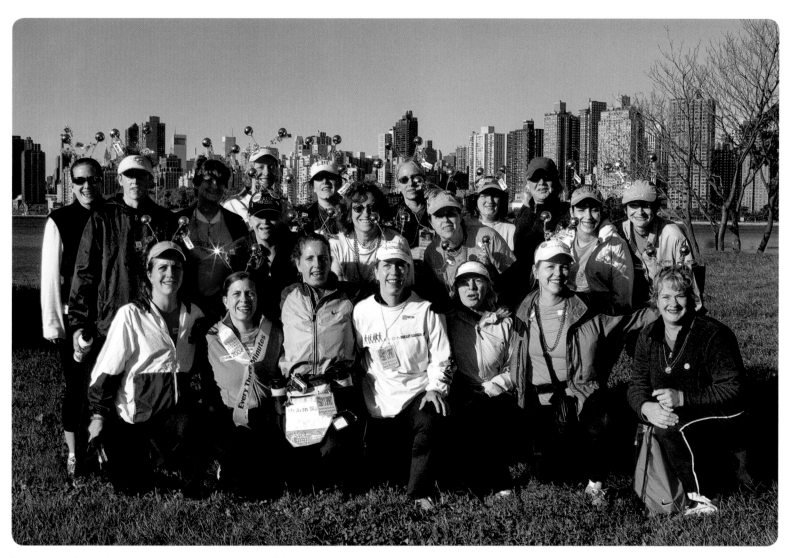

heavyset, but they were all going to walk 60 miles. It was amazing. I decided I had to be around these people."

For the 2002 event in New York, the team expanded to 11 members—including Mike, four of his sisters, one of his nieces, and a number of friends. Peggy's Spirit walked 20 miles the first day, says Mike, and then, when the event was canceled because of bad weather, the team walked on its own the next two days.

In 2003, Mike represented Peggy's Spirit at the Avon Walks in New York, Boston, and Chicago. He was just hitting his stride. He was there for all six Avon Walks in 2004, accompanied by a growing legion of Peggy's Spirit team members in Chicago, Los Angeles, and New York. At the final event, in New York, Mike reports that the team swelled to 35 members, including six of Peggy's daughters, two nieces, a cousin, a daughter-in-law, and "a great bunch of my sisters' friends." Other family members served as crew members and volunteers. For the whole year, says Mike, Peggy's Spirit contributed $115,000 to the Avon Walk for Breast Cancer series.

If his commitment seems remarkable, Mike has a simple rationale: "It has to be done, and I'm able to do it." This is the right fight at the right time, and Mike intends to be part of it. He is also confident that the battle will be won, that the cure is coming, and that when a cure for one cancer is found, "it will explode across the line" and lead to the end of all cancers. Maybe it will be the team of scientists at the American Cancer Society, or "maybe a researcher like I met up in Boston who is working his buns off 16 hours a day all by himself," says Mike, "but I know it's going to happen, and I'm going to be there to see it—God willing."

By strange coincidence, both Mike and his sister Kathleen had the same unforgettable experience at different 2004 Avon Walk events. He in Chicago and she in New York were among the walkers chosen to wear the special pink "EVERY THREE MINUTES" ribbon—with its terrible reminder that a new breast cancer diagnosis occurs every three minutes. Both consider it one of the most emotionally difficult things they've ever been asked to do. As

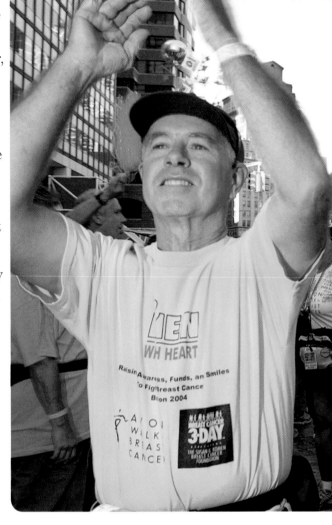

Kathleen explains, "I had five sisters with me, a brother, a sister-in-law, cousins, lifelong friends, and the fear of this disease suddenly became so personal. It convinced me that this must come to an end. That's why we're doing this— to bring an end to breast cancer."

The force pushing toward a cure, says Mike, is awareness, and the more people walking at each event, the more awareness is raised. One of Mike's donors, an oncology nurse, told him of a woman "who walked into the doctor's office with breasts bruised like rotten oranges." At that point, says Mike, there was nothing they could do. "Why didn't she come earlier? Why didn't she examine herself? So we are walking to wake people up." The money raised

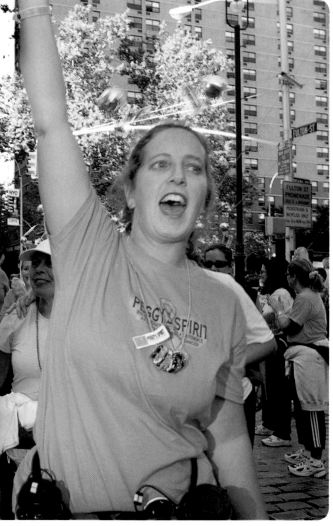

is critical, obviously, but it's the throngs of people that get the attention. "If I had gone out and raised $11,000 and just walked in one event, the financial impact would have been the same," he explains, "but the numbers matter just as much. It's important for us to get out there as often as possible and make ourselves visible."

As a man walking for a cause so closely associated with women, Mike says he has taken special inspiration from another man he met at the Avon Walk in Boston—a man named Bill, in his late 50s, who had had both knees replaced. When Mike caught up with him on Saturday, Bill was walking alone, near the back of the pack, moving in painfully tiny steps "like a baby who has just found his legs." Bill told Mike he was determined to walk 13 miles on Saturday and another 13 on Sunday. When Mike asked him why, Bill responded, "My wife and her girlfriend are up there in front of the crowd, and they believe in this cause. And I'm here because I believe in my wife." Mike says that was all he needed to hear. "Bill reminded me of how so many men are: we believe in our women, but we don't always show it." What better way to show it than to take up arms in the battle against breast cancer?

Mike gives thanks that none of his sisters have had breast cancer, and he rejoices even more when he sees them participating in these events. As he points out, all that walking, in and of itself, is a sure path to good health. "You better believe they are taking care of themselves," he says. "That exercise, the training miles, the stretching— these things have extraordinary benefits. You keep your heart pumping, your muscles toned; you're doing marvelous things for your body."

Mike's own body will be reaping those benefits—in spades. He has signed up to participate in all eight Avon Walks scheduled for 2005. Beyond that, he plans to keep at it "until this disease has been beaten." Mike says he knows "too many women who have been lost or who are suffering unnecessarily. Women have suffered enough from breast cancer."

If Mike and his family have anything to do with it, "Peggy's Spirit" will prevail.

Sharon Forbes & Karen Cannuta
Washington, D.C.

"You're missing a big piece of why you're on earth if you have not done something like this." —*Karen Cannuta*

Hi! We're Sharon and Karen —two sisters walking in memory of our mother, Shirley, who died on May 14, 2004, from a rare and very aggressive form of metastatic kidney cancer. She loved to travel, loved giving homes to homeless animals, and loved making sure that, even when the seasons might not change according to schedule, her garden did.

Throughout her life, our mom wouldn't dream of letting the prospect of an adventure pass her by, and that usually meant we went along for the ride. We're sure she wouldn't miss out on something this big, so we *know* she'll be with us along the way!

Our mom was a *very* special, *very* amazing person—and so are you for what you're doing here at the 3-Day. We hope you have an inspiring journey and bring home thousands of special memories . . . one for each step of the way.

Enjoy the walk and stay dry!

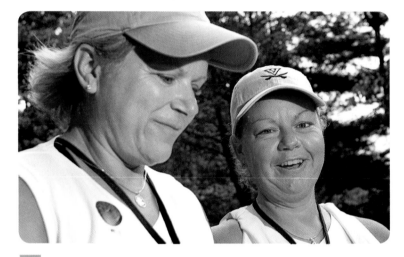

This was the message that Sharon Forbes and Karen Cannuta handed out to more than 1,000 of their fellow walkers at the Breast Cancer 3-Day Walk in Washington, D.C. Along with the yellow slips of paper, the sisters handed out bright, beautiful, yellow sunflowers, and therein lies a story.

"It was just a couple of days before Mom died," says Sharon. "It had not been easy. She had been in great pain, and it was really very difficult for her to communicate with us. I told her we needed to come up with a plan." There had to be a way, Sharon felt, for her mother to let the family know that, once she passed over, everything was okay. Because their mother was an avid gardener, it occurred to Sharon that the "code word" would be sunflowers. "I told her, 'You

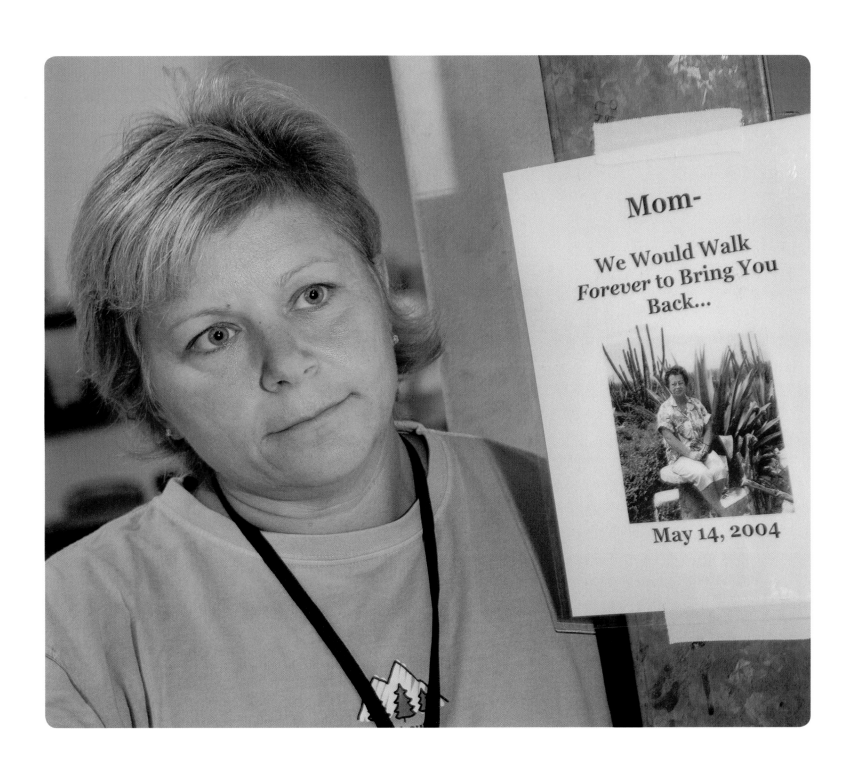

The poster reads:

Mom-

We Would Walk Forever to Bring You Back...

May 14, 2004

know, just out of the blue, just let me see some sunflowers. I'll know they're from you, a message that you're okay.'"

The day after her mom died, Sharon got a "junk e-mail" from a florist she had never heard of. "It was a huge bouquet of sunflowers with a message that said, 'Sunflowers say I love you and have a nice day.' Karen and I couldn't believe it."

It was also shortly before their mother died that Sharon and Karen decided to walk in her honor at the Breast Cancer 3-Day. As Karen put it, "We wanted to let people know about Mom's story because she was a very independent, strong woman. She loved adventure, loved going down roads she had never been through before. So this was a three-day adventure that, spiritually, we would all be on together. We just wanted to make sure people knew about our mom."

As so often happens, the walk also gave the sisters a chance to put their experience with their mother, and their own sorrow, into a larger perspective. "You really get a chance to walk in other people's shoes for a while," says Sharon, "and there aren't many opportunities in this life to do that. Hearing other people's stories is to me probably the most important thing to take away from the experience."

Karen says that on the second day, when she was really "starting to whine," starting to wonder why in the world her sister got her into this, starting to worry about nothing except all the blisters on her feet, she struck up a conversation with a survivor. "This woman was telling me about her mastectomy and her reconstructive surgery and everything she had been through, and it made me realize, 'Walking is nothing. This is a piece of cake.'" Karen says there are lots of things she can't do. She's not a doctor; she's not going to be the one to find a cure. "But I have two good legs. I have a brain. I have a mouth. I can spread the word, I can convince people to give, and I can keep my mother's memory alive." She can also "remind people of what's important in life," she says, "because we have so many distractions."

It didn't matter to Sharon and Karen that their mother had died of renal cancer rather than breast cancer, and it didn't matter to anyone else either. "That makes no difference," says Karen. "The point is that you are doing something to help another person or another family. Whatever kind of cancer it is, you still have to go through the same things, the same emotions—like just hearing the words, 'You have cancer.'"

Karen calls the experience of the walk "awesome, unforgettable"—particularly the complete absence of any negative vibration. "If someone stopped to tie their shoe, it was like, 'Are you okay? Do you need anything?' It didn't matter what you look like; nobody cares how big you are, how fat, how skinny, how pretty, how ugly. The only thing that mattered was everybody getting together to do this one good thing. I didn't know what that could feel like in such a big way, and it was totally incredible to me. I mean, I have never felt the power of women like I felt those three days."

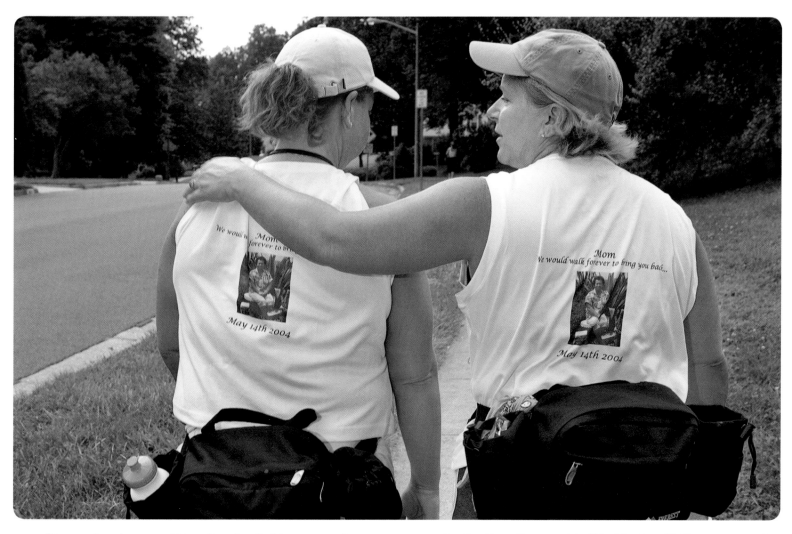

Sharon has been walking for charitable causes for several years. Karen, having now done it for the first time, can't believe what she's been missing. "This is something everybody must experience," she says. "You don't become totally human, I don't think, or you're missing a big piece of why you are here on earth if you have not done something like this."

By the time the event in Washington, D.C., was over, the sisters had made plans to walk together at the 3-Day Walk in Boston. They're already working out the sunflower logistics.

As Sharon says, "To have a thousand people walking around with sunflowers . . . well, Mom was always a very private person, and this is our way of giving her her 15 minutes."

Karen, Danielle, & Brittany Cook

Washington, D.C.

"Walking across that finish line, with all those people cheering you on, was the most amazing experience ever." —Karen Cook

Karen, the oldest of the three Cook sisters, was 13 when her mother died of breast cancer in 1994. Danielle was 11, and Brittany was only 7. Even Karen, whose eighth-grade school year began the day her mother passed away, "had basically never heard of breast cancer" at the time, and her sisters were even less aware of what was happening.

Ten years later, Karen decided that the time had come for the sisters to get involved in the fight against breast cancer—and at the same time to commemorate their mother's life. "I wanted to do something *big*," says Karen. "Raising $2,000 and walking 60 miles would definitely be a challenge. It was something I really wanted to do."

Brittany, by then a 17-year-old high schooler, needed no convincing. "It was, 'Sounds great. When are we going?'" says

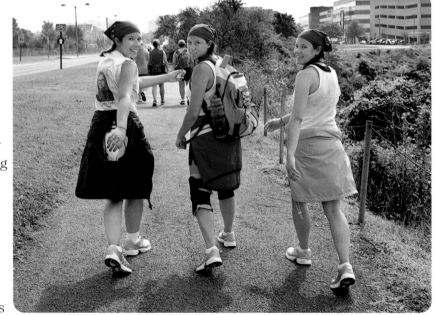

Karen. Danielle, busy with college life and a job as well, wasn't so sure, until Karen did the big-sister thing. "Finally I just had to tell her, 'Hey, you're coming up here and doing this with us.' Then she was like, 'Okay.'"

For these three young women—a recent college graduate, a college student, and a high school student—fundraising was not going to be easy. Karen took the lead. "I was consumed with it," she says. She distributed flyers to every place she could think of, wrote letters to every family member she knew (and asked them to appeal to everybody *they* knew), and hosted a Ben & Jerry's night, among other things.

Their father was standing by, slightly skeptical that the girls could pull it off. "I told him to have a little faith," says Karen. When it was all said and done, Dad contributed "maybe $200" and the

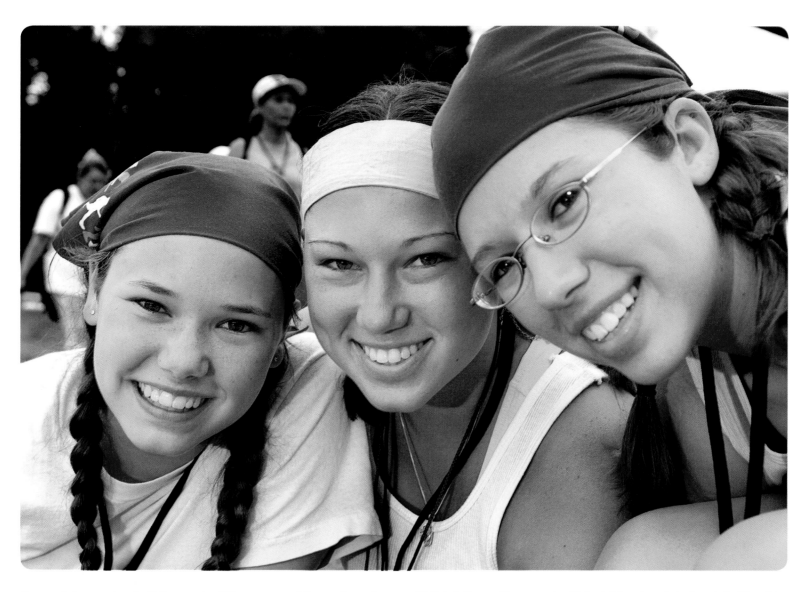

three sisters raised all the rest of the money. Karen found out what so many others have learned in fundraising for these events: "I guess people just wanted to give."

If the fundraising was easier than they expected, the walk itself was harder. "I was definitely hurting," says Karen. "I think I was the worst off, but I kept quiet about it. I had to practically crawl across the finish line." Her sisters weren't doing much better. Danielle had brought braces for both knees but had to give one to Brittany. As Karen describes it, "They were both kind of hobbling there toward the end."

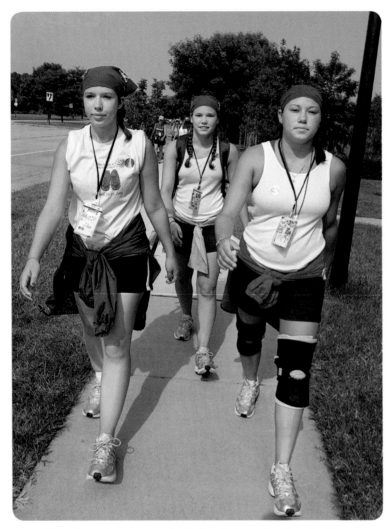

endless miles of sidewalk still to be covered. "There was still such a *long, long* way to go," says Karen, when suddenly they noticed a church looming directly ahead. "It was St. Bernadette's Cathedral, and all three of us just, like, stopped in our tracks. Our mother's name is Bernadette." They had no idea there was such a church in the area, but none of them doubted the significance of seeing it. "It was a sign," says Karen. "She was there with us. It was the motivation we needed to make it the rest of the way."

Karen says that the best thing about the walk was that it gave the sisters a chance to reunite for those three days. "We've always been close, but we had not spent time together like that for a while. The difficulty of the walk and the emotions of the occasion really brought us together." Most important, she says, was the chance they had to talk about their mother, "to remember things about her," and to share their feelings about what had happened to her.

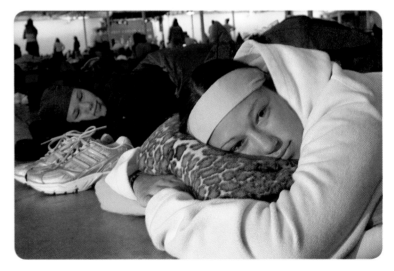

Two knee braces and all the determination in the world might still not have been enough, had not the sisters also received one of those almost miraculous moments of inspiration when they needed it the most. It was on the third day, Karen recalls, when they were physically beat and emotionally drained. They had just emerged from a wooded area along the route and were looking ahead at what seemed

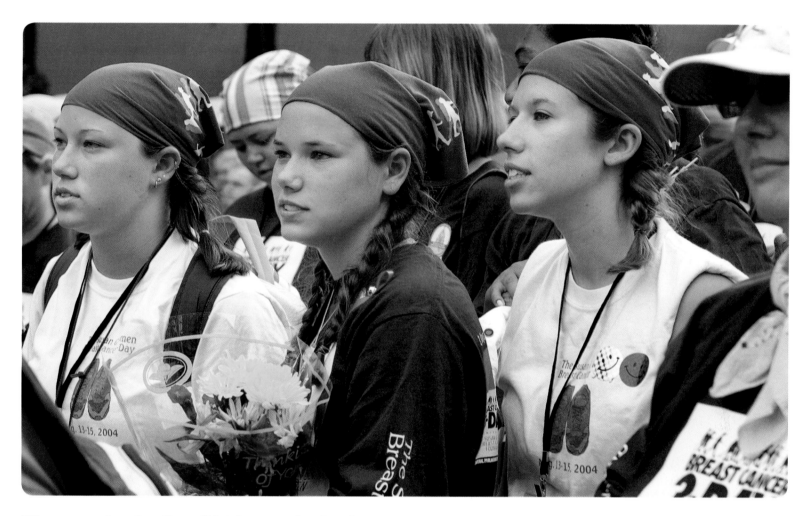

"There was a lot of stuff we didn't know at the time," says Karen, "and hadn't really ever talked about. It was time to talk about all those things."

Karen also appreciates how the walk—and other such events—raises awareness of breast cancer and the pervasive threat it poses. "They tell women to get a mammogram when they turn 40," she notes, "but Mom died when she was 39. These events make you realize that it can happen to you."

The good news is that seeing the huge crowds that turn out for these events makes you realize that times are changing. "When I was 13," says Karen, "I had never heard of breast cancer. I guarantee you that that couldn't happen today. You see all these people and you know there's a reason why they're here. You realize something needs to be done about this disease—and that something *is* being done."

Walking in
Spirit

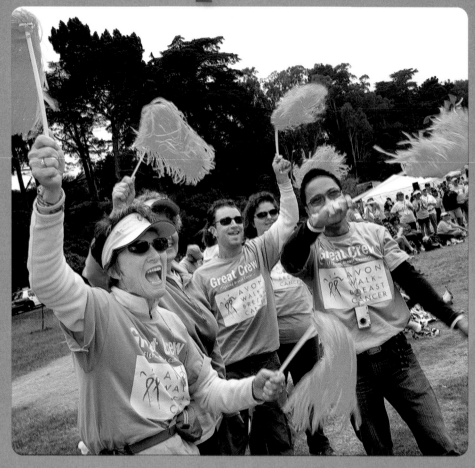

Walkers have support from friends and family when they sign up for the event, but what many of them don't know is that they will have a whole new family supporting them behind the scenes. These are the people who feed them, cheer them, provide medical assistance, help set up their tents, and hand out water. They are "the crew," and their stories are often as moving as the walkers'. A husband might crew while his survivor-wife walks; a family might crew together in memory of their mom; people might simply crew to be part of a great cause. Whatever their reasons, the events could not happen without them.

I walk because...

"The walk is the best place for the caregivers to learn, too. Breast cancer is not just about the person who has it; it affects everyone in his or her life. But the caregivers don't know what to say; they don't know what to do. Participating in one of the walks changes all that. You learn so fast how to support your loved one." —*Tim Day*

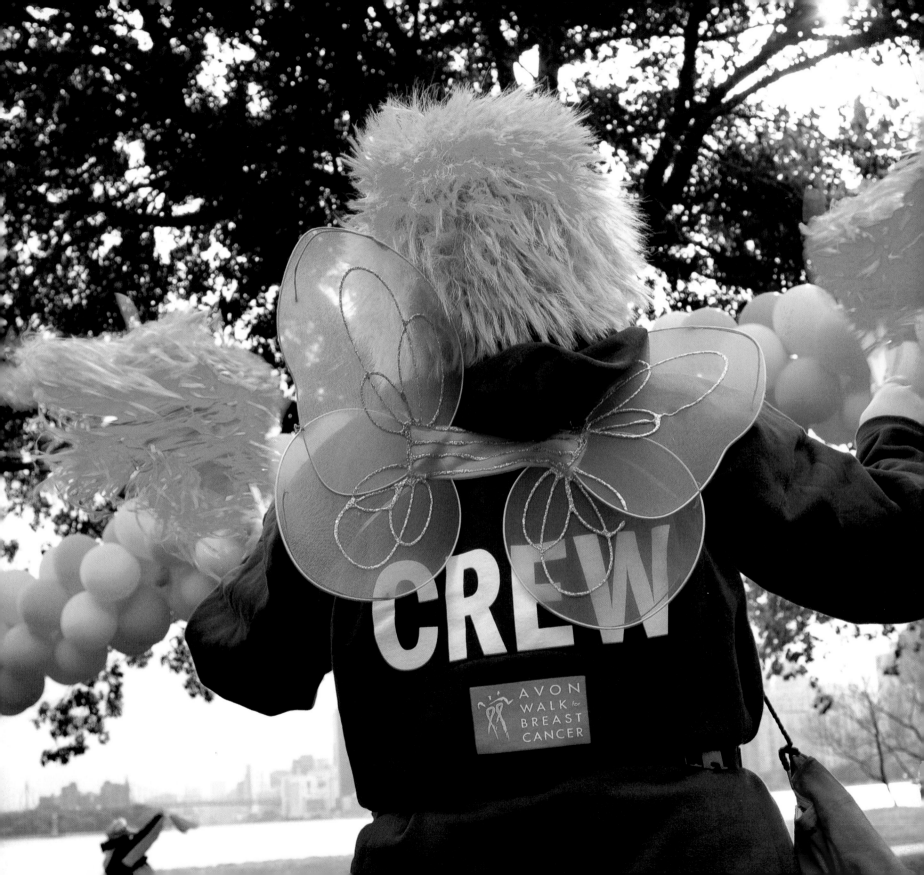

The Ammon Family

Ashburn, Virginia

"We wanted to crew because the walkers need people to help them raise those millions of dollars. It was a fantastic experience." —Craig Ammon

The Ammon family got involved in the fight against breast cancer after Steve's wife and the mother of his three children died of the disease in 2001. As son Craig explains, it was really his mother and father's long-time friend, Mary Jo, who gave them the impetus. She had already participated in several breast cancer walks in memory of her sister, and when she signed up to walk again in 2002, Steve decided to walk with her in his wife's memory. One by one the children registered for the event as well.

"First my sister, Kelly, signed up, then my brother, Chris, and meanwhile I'm thinking, *How in the world am I going to raise $2,000, especially when they've already hit up all of our mutual friends?*"

It was a real challenge, says Craig, but he raised the money, and the whole gang—Steve and Mary Jo, Kelly, Craig, and Chris—joined together in the Avon Breast Cancer 3-Day in 2002.

It was an unforgettable experience—"a wonderful time bonding with my family"—but, for Craig, it wasn't enough. Even then, at his first breast cancer event in 2002, he saw what he really wanted to be doing. In the first

place, says Craig, "my style has always been working behind the scenes and helping people out." When he saw the crew members "running around helping people with their tents in the pouring rain and getting up early and serving breakfast with a big smile for everybody," Craig says he was "just really envious."

Then there's the fact that because everybody walks at a different pace, even when you're trying to interact with the other walkers "you're still only going to see a hundred or so walkers at the most." For Craig, that didn't compare to being able to serve breakfast and offer a cheerful "Good morning" to all 4,500. Crewing, Craig concluded, "just seemed like a really cool thing to do."

How does a person turn out to be so generous and considerate and kind? The answer emerges when Craig talks about his "awesome" mother, a woman who "always made sure her children appreciated the gifts they had and were grateful for their opportunities." Around the Ammon house, there was no griping about "another day of work." Instead, it was "Thank God I can put my feet on the ground and get up and go to work, because there are plenty of people who can't."

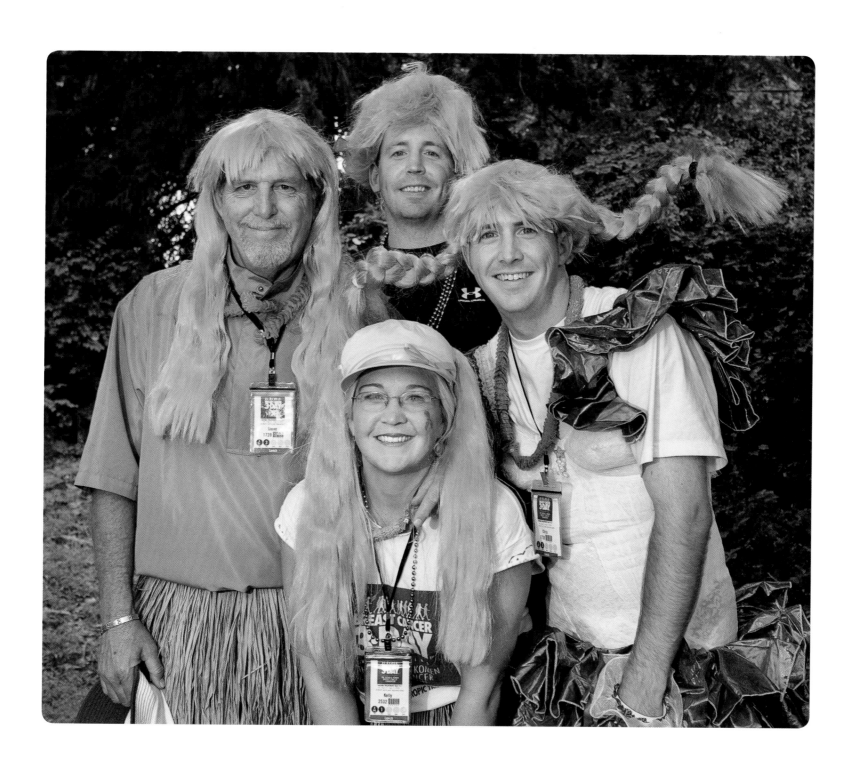

Craig says his mom was first diagnosed in 1980, when Kelly, the oldest, was 14, Craig was 12, and Chris was 9. "We really couldn't spare her income at the time," says Craig, and, of course, the three children couldn't spare her from their lives. "So she would do things like go to chemo in the morning, go home and have a nap, go to work in the afternoon, then pick me up for swim practice. It must have been so hard, but she really tried not to miss a beat."

His mother was cancer-free for 17 years, says Craig, but even when she was diagnosed again in 1997, "she continued to be as upbeat as she possibly could." Her spirit was such that Craig and Chris were sure that the chemo was doing its job and that they would have her with them for many more years. "That was what we thought six weeks before she died," says Craig, "because that was the story she had us believing."

Craig says his mother was just "an incredibly strong person and our biggest cheerleader throughout school and sports and college." Therein lies the connection: Craig's mom would have loved being a crew member. "You know, getting up early to get ready for the pit stops, setting up the camp, high-fiving the walkers, cheering and acting crazy and stuff like that—that's just the epitome of what my mom was."

In 2003 Craig and his father took the plunge, and in 2004 the whole family crewed together at the Breast Cancer 3-Day Walk in Washington. Not surprisingly, they took the experience to the limits, as evidenced by the hi-

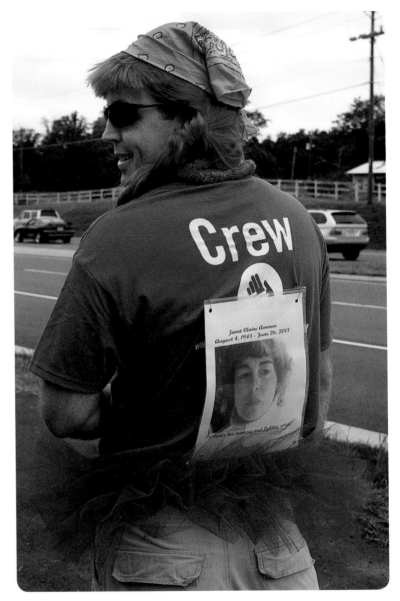

larious outfits they wore—gaudy wigs, grass skirts, tutus, the works. Actually, says Craig, it wasn't their idea to wear women's costumes. Their crew chief had brought all the attire, assuming that, as in previous years, the lunch crew would be all female. The Ammon men didn't blink. In fact, says Craig, there was a bit of sibling rivalry to see who could make their outfit look the wackiest. "We got sort of psyched up that night—getting everything ready to go at four a.m."

Craig says the weekend's special moment for him came at breakfast on Day Two when he sat down to talk to a woman who was eating breakfast by herself. She told Craig she was hurting from Day One but was determined to finish and "prove all her coworkers wrong." She "teared up" when she said she

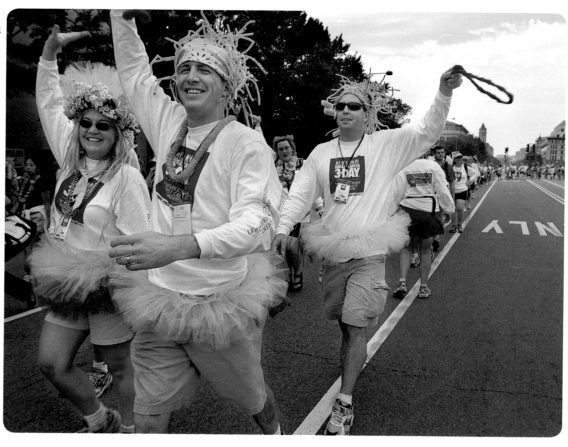

was walking in memory of her mother, who had died the previous January. Craig consoled her by saying that she was where he had been two years earlier, and that her mother would be so proud of her. "She said her mother would probably think she was as crazy as her father thought she was," recalls Craig, "and I thought, *Wow, this poor woman's got everybody against her.*" Craig says the woman was a little overweight, and he could just imagine that "physically and emotionally it was going to be a struggle for her." He says he cheered her on at lunch that day

and looked for her on Day Three. "I didn't see her till the end, but then saw her crossing the finish line hand-in-hand with a group of other women, then saw them all laughing and high-fiving everybody. To have met her two days and 40 miles earlier, and then to see her reach her goal—that was a real high point for me."

Right before the event, by the way, Steve married Mary Jo. He returned from the honeymoon just in time. "To have him back working with the three of us for those three straight days," says Craig, "was just very cool."

Phil & Lynne Hall

San Francisco, California

"I came to realize that the more I make them smile, the less pain they're in while they're walking." —Phil Hall

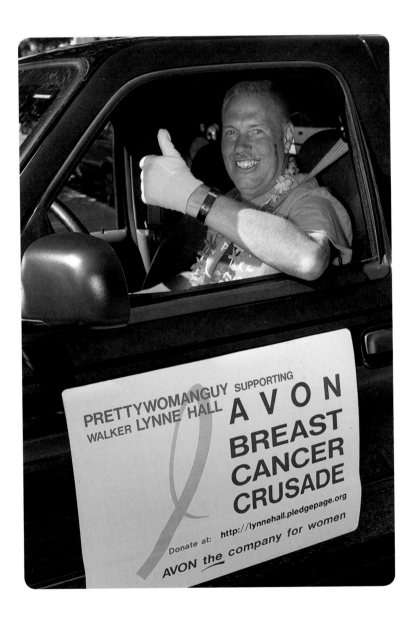

Lynne Hall might demur if you called her "Pretty Woman." But there's no question that her husband, Phil, is "Pretty Woman Man."

Their journey toward these identities began in January 1999, when Lynne's annual mammogram showed something that "looked suspicious." Actually, she had had a lump for some time before that, but it had been dismissed as a cyst. "They told me not to worry about it," Lynne says, but she did worry in 1999 when she was called back in for a needle biopsy. She was so worried, in fact, that she told the doctor to call Phil with the results. "I didn't know how I would handle it," Lynne recalls, "so Phil got the phone call. Then he called me and asked if I could take a break from work and meet him, which told me what the news was."

"We grew a lot closer during that conversation," says Phil, who understood immediately how important his support was going to be. "A lot of husbands go straight into denial," he says. "But when a woman gets this diagnosis, she needs support and she needs help. She needs companionship. This is not the time to run away. That message needs to get out there."

So when Lynne decided to participate in the Avon Breast Cancer 3-Day in 2001, Phil knew he would be there,

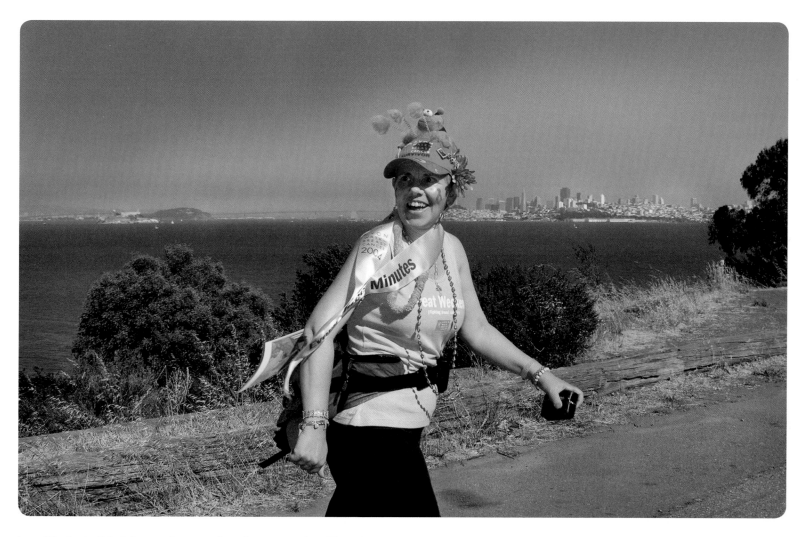

too. He just didn't know in exactly what capacity. Then he heard the rumor: some guy in a convertible with "Pretty Woman" playing on the radio had driven by a training walk, and all the women had gotten a big kick out of it. So he made himself a CD that played "Pretty Woman" 25 times and showed up at the event. "I was planning to play it for my wife at the beginning of the walk when everybody was coming out of the convention center," says Phil, "then maybe wait for her again at another part of the walk. So there I was, playing the song really loud in my pickup truck, cheering and yelling for my wife. But then I realized that there were thousands of walkers coming out, just rows and rows of them walking by, so I decided I'd better stay there and cheer them all on." Pretty Woman Man was born.

And as for the pink glove that has become a Pretty Woman Man trademark? "Well," says Phil, "that first day I clapped until my hand was bloody raw, so the next day I got a work glove out of my truck and yelled and cheered

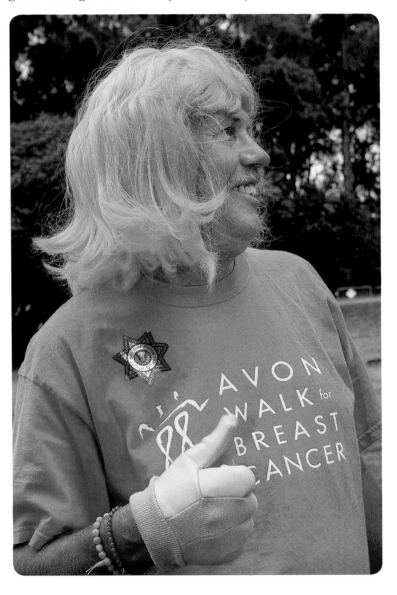

and clapped some more. It got to be part of the bargain: you walk and get blisters on your feet, and I clap and get blisters on my hand. Since then the work glove has evolved into a pink cotton gardening glove."

Meanwhile, that first year Lynne had an experience that she says was almost too incredible to describe. "The excitement of the event and all the people involved just carries you through," says Lynne. "You feel a sense of belonging not only with the group of women you train with but with the whole 'walk community'—including the people who come out to support us. It's difficult to put into words the feeling you have after participating in something like this."

Lynne says she walked the whole 60 miles and immediately wanted to sign up for the next year's event, but she wasn't sure how Phil would feel about that. "Phil said, 'How can we not?' He can't pull away from it because of how it makes him feel and how wonderful he thinks all the walkers are."

In fact, Lynne has walked—with Phil cheering—every year since 2001, for the past two years as part of a team called the "Warming Hut Hotties." Lynne explains that the team's organizer thought that by pulling a group together she could better motivate herself to train and walk, so she started putting the word out. "At the first meeting," says Lynne, "six people showed up. The next weekend, a few more, and it just kept growing from there." Lynne isn't sure exactly how they came up with that name, but the Warming Hut at San Francisco's Crissy Field is where they meet for the training walks. She does know that the team now has more than 100 members and has raised a whole lot of money.

Leave it to Pretty Woman Man, the team's unofficial recruiter, to have the exact figures: "The Warming Hut Hotties set a record for the number of walkers—it's the largest group in the U.S., with 118 members. This year we raised $321,747, which also makes us the largest fundraising group."

Neither Lynne nor Phil shows any inclination to drop out of the vanguard. For Lynne, it's partly a matter of the "pride and satisfaction" to be derived from being part of "such a fantastic cause." But it's more than that. "You just keep meeting more and more wonderful people who are involved in this," she explains. "Not just team-mates, either. Sometimes I'll just strike up a conversation with a stranger and learn what their story is and why they are walking. It's so powerful, so incredible. It's contagious. It's a life-altering experience."

If it's contagious, Phil is a vector. He says he was on-line looking for some feedback to the whole Pretty Woman Man thing, and found a woman who wrote, "First it was cute. Then it was annoying. Then it was necessary." After reading that, says Phil, "How can I stop?"

Phil says he has to stay on the sidelines because he has trouble walking. But that's okay. The women can count on Pretty Woman Man. "I really believe that whether you have that support or not can make the difference between winning or losing the fight."

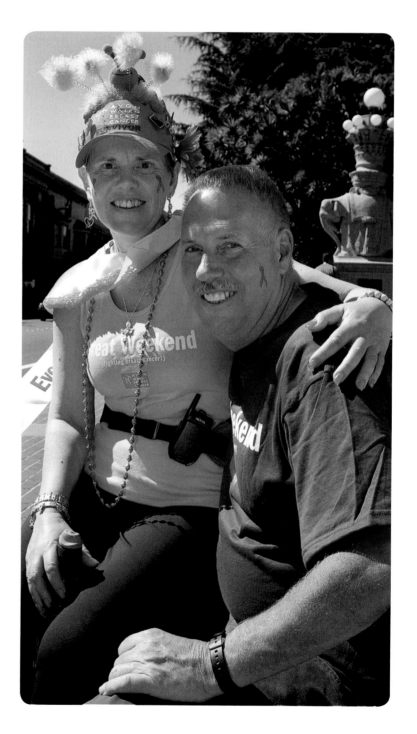

Encouragement

It's amazing what a smile, a silly costume, or a high five can do to get you over the hump when your feet are killing you and your brain says, "I'm done." The cheerleaders might be kids handing out candy, crew members, "Pretty Woman Man," or friends waiting on the side of the road with signs and balloons. What a lift it is to hear "Thanks for walking!" or "You're almost there!" A cool spray of water from a garden hose can be just the thing to get you up that hill.

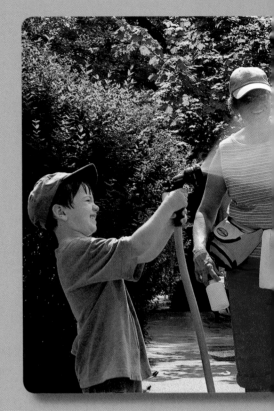

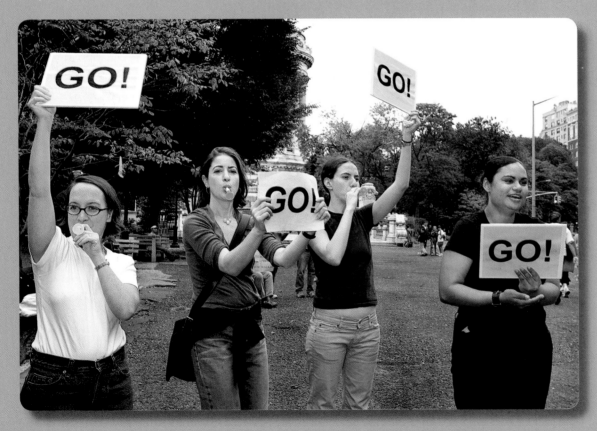

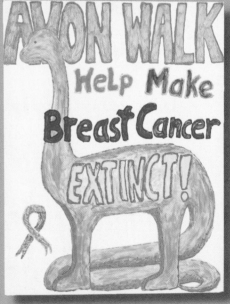

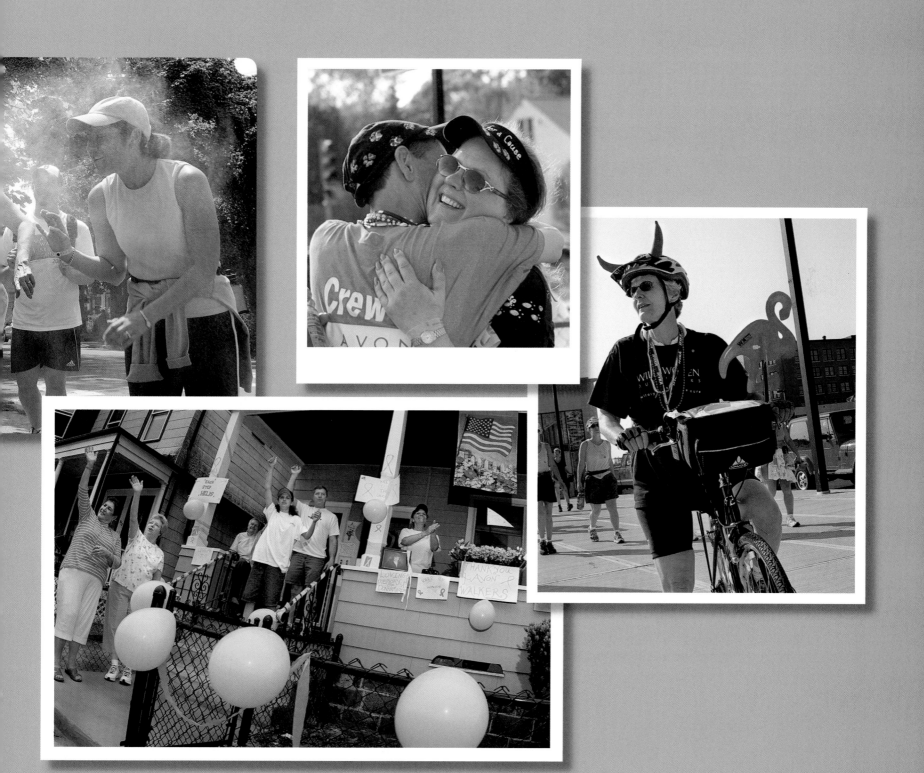

Jim Bezy
Warren, Michigan

"I sure hope I brightened the walkers' day a little bit because they sure brightened mine—even in the rain."

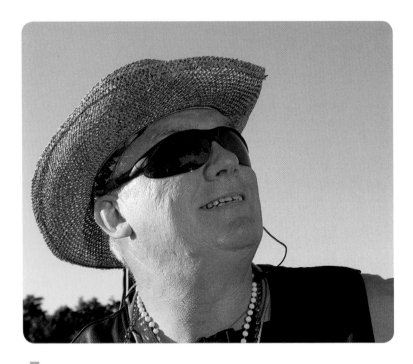

Jim Bezy's "beloved wife" of 27 years died of breast cancer on November 2, 2002. She had been diagnosed in 1995, just after her 43rd birthday, with stage 4 metastatic cancer. "She was given about one year to live," says Jim, "which is a pretty harsh sentence." The doctor told her, though, that she had to see herself as part of that 18 percent who survive. "If you want to fight, you've got to commit to it," he told Ella, and Ella said, "I'm committing to it." She survived seven years.

"We tried to live every minute," says Jim, "and not waste one moment of time being angry or upset about things we couldn't control. We just wanted to live our lives and hope that they would come up with a cure. I mean, that's everybody's dream, that they will find a cure and you can keep on living your life. That wasn't to be, but seven years, to me, was a gift."

When a neighbor who knew Jim's story mentioned that the Breast Cancer 3-Day was coming to Detroit, Jim saw a way to be part of that effort to find a cure. "She knew I had a motorcycle," says Jim, "and that another neighbor, Roger, also had a bike. She said that they had a route safety crew and thought I might want to participate." Talking to Roger about it later, Jim found out that his sister-in-law had died of breast cancer some years before and that his wife and daughter had been on the medical crew "and just loved it." Jim jumped at the chance to get involved. (Crew members, by the way, are not asked to raise money, but Jim raised $1,800 anyway.)

If you've ever participated in a breast cancer walk and wondered if the "route safety crew" receives any instruction, the answer, basically, is no. As Jim explains, "Pretty much all they told us was 'make big motions with

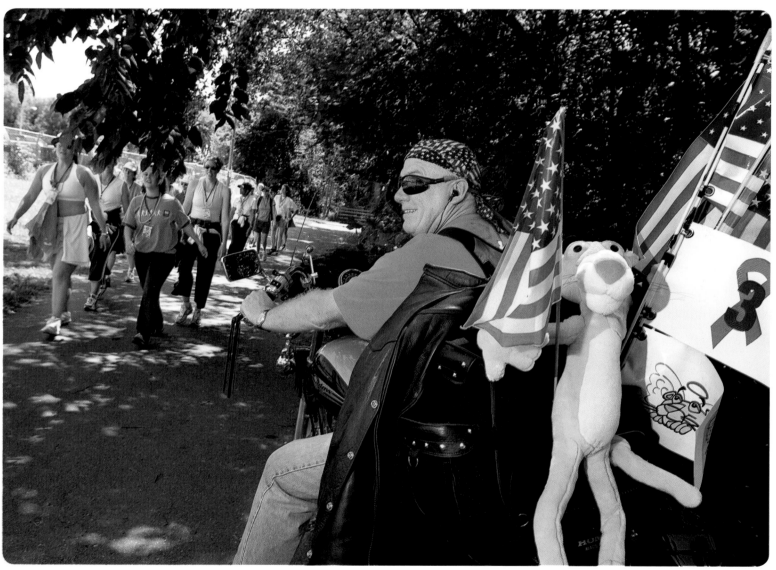

your hands,' since people in cars are kind of oblivious to walkers." As for rules, Jim says, they were given three: "First was to keep ourselves safe. Second was to keep all the walkers safe. Third was to have fun. I think we accomplished all three."

Just about the first thing Jim noticed, once he was on the job, was the incredible marketing savvy of Harley-Davidson. "All the women kept saying, 'Hey, can I sit on your Harley and get a picture?' or 'Hey, I love your Harley.' Everybody seems to think that all motorcycles are Harleys."

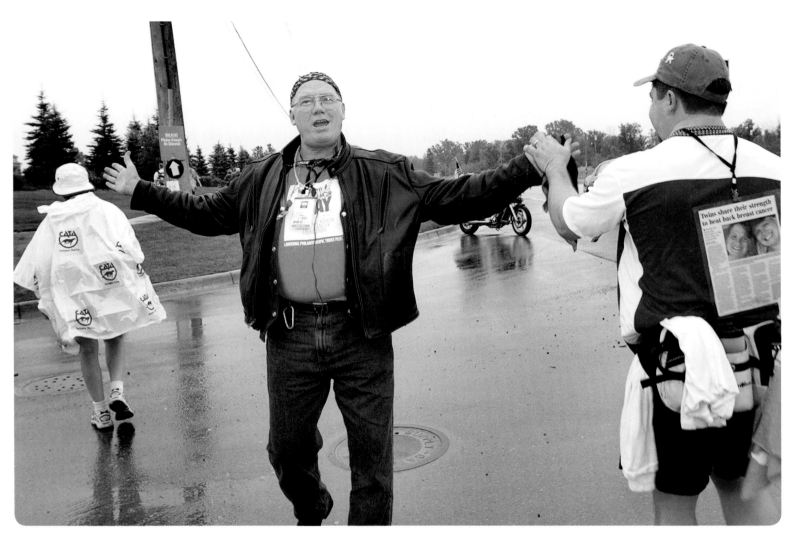

In fact, says Jim, of the eight motorcycles in the route safety crew, half were Hondas, including his. But if the walkers got a lift by sitting on his "Harley," that was fine with Jim.

More accurately, says Jim, it was the walkers who gave him a lift, and very soon he found himself high-fiving them all as they passed by. "They were so amazing. I told them, 'You ladies are just inspiring the heck out of us,' and then they would say, 'No, you guys are inspiring us to keep walking.'" But as Jim points out, they were the ones walking 60 miles, which was farther than he'd ever walked even in the army. "I was honored," says Jim, "to be there helping these women who were really committed to doing something so positive. You couldn't help but encourage them to press on."

Jim says he will cherish many memories from the event—the "Cowgirls from Texas" in their pink hats and pink hot pants who had come all the way to Michigan; the husband and wife team on the safety crew who pedaled all day on bicycles, in spite of the fact that the husband had an artificial leg—but he was moved the most by the closing ceremonies. "When the survivors came in and everyone knelt down, I could so easily picture my wife in that group. It was so powerful it just gave me a chill."

Ultimately, though, Jim believes that the true meaning of the event lies in the spirit of kindness, goodwill, and hope that touches the hearts of everyone who participates. "You hear it all the time at the pit stops and breaks, people saying, 'Don't you wish the world could be like this all the time? Why does it have to end after three days?'"

It doesn't end, as Jim realizes, because the work being done in the fight against breast cancer has its own unstoppable momentum. "When people get hit with this terrible news," says Jim, "it's like getting run over by a Mack truck, but as soon as you realize that there really is hope, that people do survive, it makes you stronger."

More than anything, says Jim, events like this remind people "that a support network is out there"—and that hearing the words *You have cancer* is not a death sentence after all: "Medicine is advancing, they are finding answers, treatments that are less painful, less horrific, and people are surviving." The important thing, says Jim, is not to let the diagnosis take your hope away.

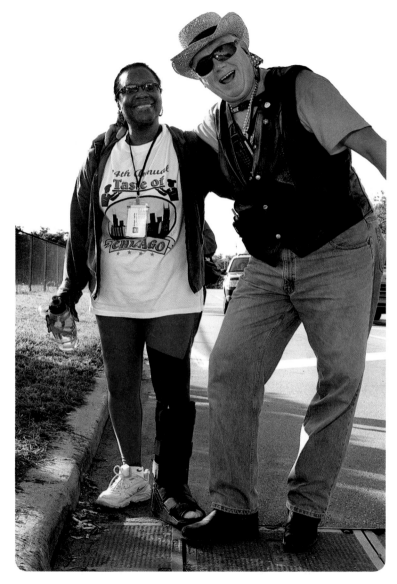

Those seven years with his beloved Ella taught Jim a deep truth: "If you're worrying about how long you've got to live your live, you never live your life. And that's the worst thing you can do. You've got to live your life."

Susan G. Komen Breast Cancer Foundation Race for the Cure®

Washington, D.C.

"We are steadfast in our faith that one day we will truly have something to celebrate: a world without breast cancer."
—*Nancy Brinker*

The fact that it was pouring down rain on that October morning in Dallas back in 1983 wasn't a problem for Susan Carter, who is now the Komen Foundation's director of communications. A reporter for the local paper at that time, she was there to cover the inaugural Komen Race for the Cure® to benefit an organization called the Susan G. Komen Foundation. Some 800 women were gathered in a mall parking lot to walk a 5K to raise money in the fight against breast cancer.

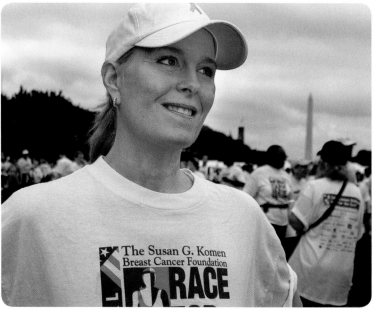

That was the problem, says Susan Carter. "I had to figure out how to write the story without using the words *breast cancer*. Back then journalists weren't comfortable using that language unless it was in a scientific context. It wasn't considered appropriate in the lifestyle or social sections of the paper, where fundraising events were traditionally covered."

Yes, indeed. We've come a long way.

Given the humble origins of the Komen Race for the Cure®, it's tempting to say that that long distance was covered on a wing and a prayer. But that's not quite the whole story. Many thousands of prayers have helped, no doubt, but for more than 20 years the Komen Foundation and its Race for the Cure Series have soared on "the power of a promise."

The Susan G. Komen Breast Cancer Foundation was founded on a very real promise made between two sisters—Susan Goodman Komen and Nancy Goodman Brinker. Suzy, as her sister called her, was diagnosed with breast cancer in 1978, a time when little was known about the disease and even less was said in public. Before she died at the age of 36, Suzy asked her sister to do everything possible to bring

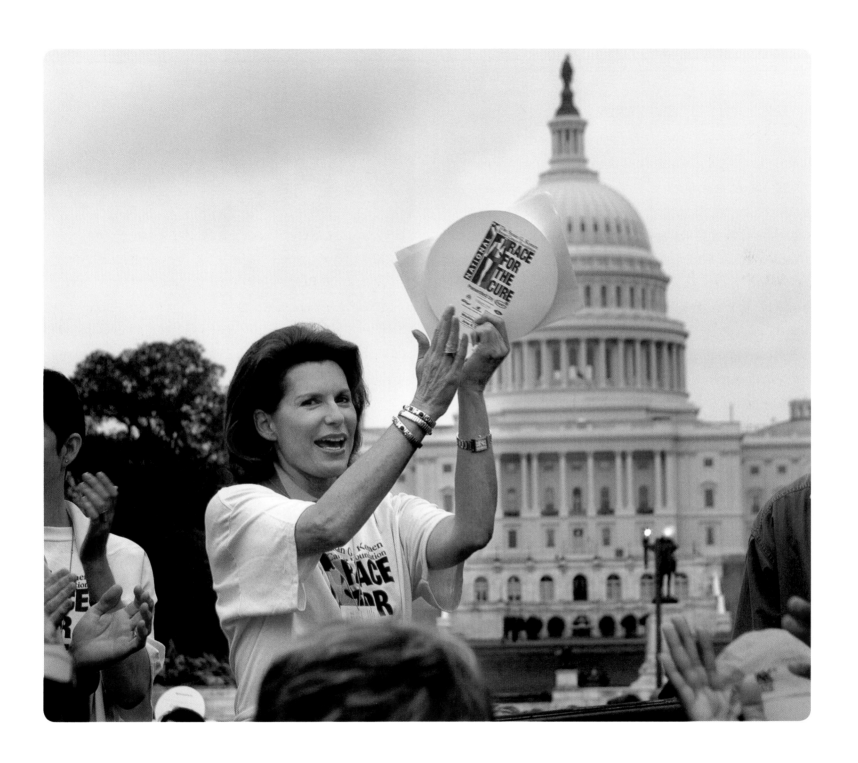

an end to breast cancer. Nancy made the promise—and has kept it. But in 1982, she wondered how she was going to.

"One of the first things Nancy wanted to do," says Susan Carter, "was to pull people together in a show of solidarity. She knew it needed to be something fun, something visual, something different to get some attention." The Komen Race for the Cure® was born. "An all-female sporting event was an entirely new concept in 1983," says Susan. "Women weren't doing too many things like that back then. The world has changed a lot."

Nancy Brinker's intuition apparently was on target. The Komen Race for the Cure® became an annual event in Dallas and quickly spread to other cities around the country. Twenty years after its inception, it's the largest series of 5K runs/fitness walks in the world—with more than one million people participating in more than 100 Race events in the U.S. as well as in Rome, Italy, and Frankfurt, Germany. As Susan Carter puts it, "The promise Nancy made to her sister has now become a promise made by millions—to bring an end to breast cancer. Everybody feels the power of the promise."

In 1990, the Komen Race for the Cure® arrived in the nation's capitol, under the title of the Susan G. Komen Breast Cancer Foundation National Race for the Cure®. The effort to bring the Race to Washington was led by former Carter White House Social Secretary Gretchen Poston and joined by Second Lady Marilyn Quayle and *Washington Post* fashion editor Nina Hyde. In that inaugural year, the

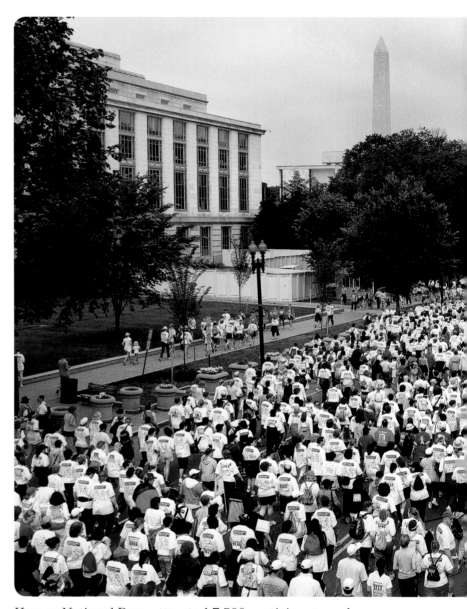

Komen National Race attracted 7,500 participants and raised more than a half million dollars. Poston herself was a breast cancer survivor and immediately set a goal for a 5K Race that would bring 25,000 runners to the streets of

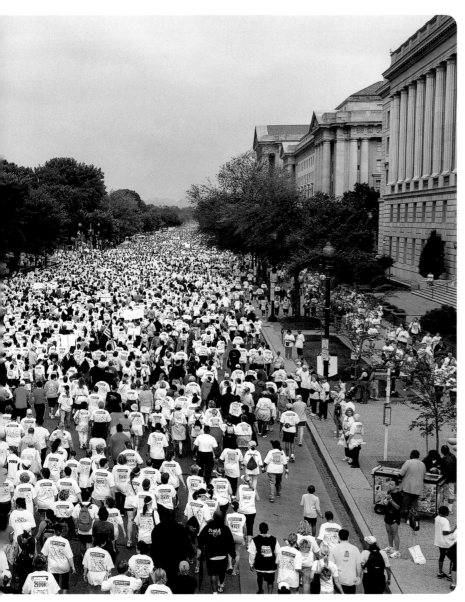

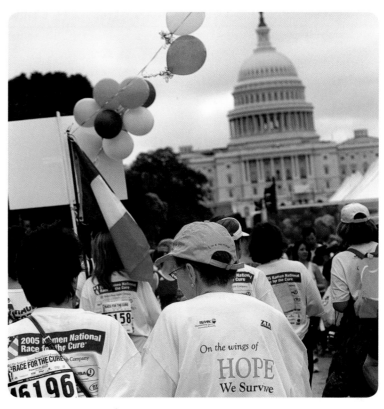

Washington and raise $1 million. In 1992, Poston lost her own courageous battle against the disease.

Since then, her dream has been more than realized. The 2004 event drew 52,000 people from all corners of the world and raised $2.5 million for breast cancer research, education, screening, and treatment.

Indeed, the Komen National Race has become one of the largest events in the Komen Foundation's signature awareness and fundraising series. Actually, says Susan Carter, the events in St. Louis and Denver draw nearly as many or more participants, with close to 60,000, but the National Race for the Cure is "a sight to see because of the venue. When you see all these people in front of the Washington Monument and all the way down the Mall, with the Capitol in the background, coming up Constitution Avenue, it's just unbelievably powerful."

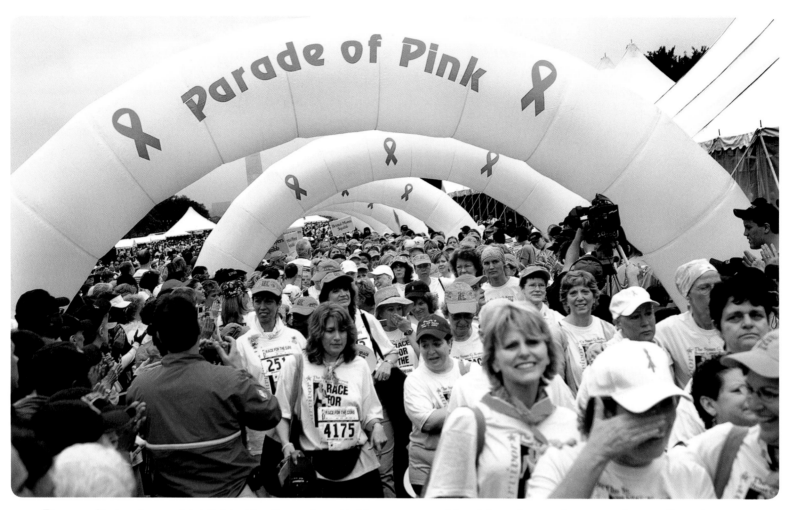

Race preliminaries are highlighted by the unforgettable "Parade of Pink"—the parade of breast cancer survivors starting at the survivor tent and ending at the bleachers. "It's just amazing," says Susan. "Nancy Brinker leads it and there are as many as 3,000 survivors participating. It's one of the largest survivor recognitions you can imagine—it just goes on forever."

One of those survivors is Magdalena Bell, who has participated in the Komen National Race for the past five years. Magdalena knew she wanted to walk, to be a part of "this great cause," but, she says, "it wasn't until I put that pink T-shirt on and became part of the pink multitude that I felt I had made the connection." Magdalena says that participating in the event brings her a deep sense of gratitude—gratitude that she's still around to tell her story. "I think all of us survivors have this inherent need to believe that the cancer is not coming back again, that we are not

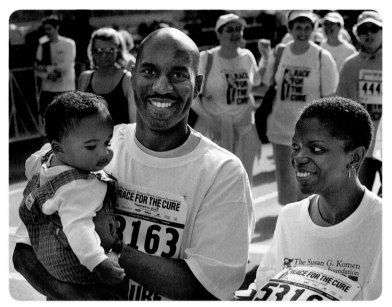

For the past two years, Magdalena has walked in the company of her two daughters, Annalese, now 13, and Alea, 17. The importance of their support, particularly after Magdalena's marriage ended, would be impossible to calculate. Annalese, who was eight when her mother was diagnosed, was too young to fully understand what Magdalena was going through. But she knew enough to make her mother get-well cards, and to keep a heart full of hope. That's what she would tell other kids, she says: "There's always hope, whether the stage is bad or the stage is good. And during the bad stage, just try to spend as much time as possible with your mother."

going to die," she says. "You really appreciate the woman who says, 'My name is Jane and I'm a 25-year survivor,' or, 'I'm Sue, and I'm a 16-year survivor.' You want that. You need that reassurance."

Set against the "majestic presence" of the nation's capitol, the experience of the Komen National Race is especially awe-inspiring, says Magdalena. She, too, like those myriad others, feels the power of the promise. "It still brings me to tears to think that this whole organization started literally on the promise from one sister to another—this organization that's now a household name. It's an international event, a part of today's vernacular: 'The Race for the Cure.' It's incredible to see the power of commitment."

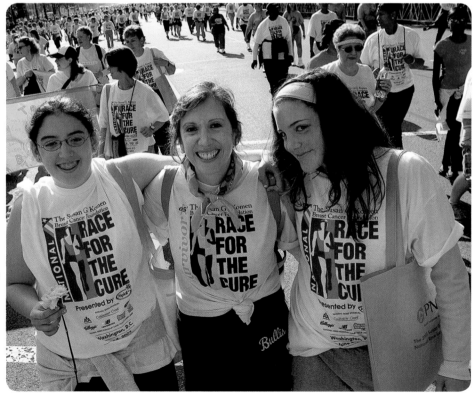

Alea says that she has always felt "a little weird" about her reaction to her mother's diagnosis. She knew that cancer was a scary thing, she says, but she never feared that Magdalena was going to die. "From the beginning, I just had this belief, this feeling that it was going to be fine." Her mother also remained very positive, says Alea, "and I think we sort of fed off of each other."

In fact, Magdalena calls her daughters "the face of the co-survivor program," a reference to one of the Komen Foundation's most far-reaching new initiatives. Launched in the spring of 2004, the program is designed to recognize the critical role played by "the people who are there" for breast cancer survivors during diagnosis, treatment, and beyond.

Susan Carter says the program was originated by two Komen Affiliates. She describes a moving scene in which all the breast cancer survivors were given a rose as they walked en masse to be recognized. They were wildly cheered on by an audience that included their co-survivors, all of whom were wearing blue T-shirts and caps. Once they had been recognized, the survivors turned to the audience and said, "Now we want to recognize all those people who have been instrumental in supporting us through our diagnosis, treatment, and recovery." With that, the survivors presented their roses to their co-survivors. "Well, there wasn't a dry eye in the house," says Susan. "It was obvious that breast cancer was truly a disease impacting the whole family and each

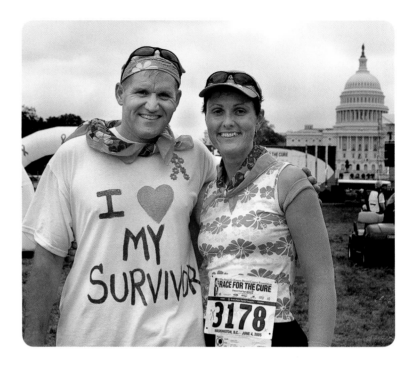

survivor drew strength from an entire support system—their co-survivors."

Susan also points out that recognizing co-survivors is not enough—which is why the program focuses on recognition *and* education. To provide the educational component, the foundation's Web site has created a special co-survivor mini-site, www.komen.org/cosurvivor, featuring useful, printable information about breast cancer; a co-survivor message board; tips and idea exchange; and a collection of real-life co-survivor stories that illustrate the program's key objectives: strength, support, and love. The Komen Foundation has also created the special pink-and-white co-survivor ribbon to signify the special relationship between a breast cancer survivor and co-survivor.

"We recognize that breast cancer is a family disease that impacts everyone—spouses, children, parents, co-workers, friends, and health care providers, and these people have their own unique challenges," says Wendy Mason, manager of the Komen Foundation's National Toll-Free Breast Care Helpline. "We believe in treating the whole patient—mind, body, and soul. When you help the co-survivor, you help the breast cancer survivor."

The final measure of the power of a promise is the fact that now, more than 20 years later, the Komen Foundation is a global leader in the fight against breast cancer. The foundation fulfills its mission through support of innovative breast cancer research grants, meritorious awards, and educational, scientific, and community outreach programs around the world. Together with its Affiliate Network of more than 75,000 volunteers, corporate partners, and generous donors, the Komen Foundation has raised more than $740 million for the fight against breast cancer.

In particular, the Komen Race for the Cure® touches people of all ages, races, and backgrounds with lifesaving messages about early detection and other breast health information. Wearing their "IN MEMORY OF" and "IN CELEBRATION OF" signs in honor of breast cancer survivors and those who have lost their battle with the disease, Race participants carry forward the most critical message: there still is a need to raise awareness about this devastating disease.

As Nancy Brinker says, much remains to be done. "We're renewing our promise in the fight against breast

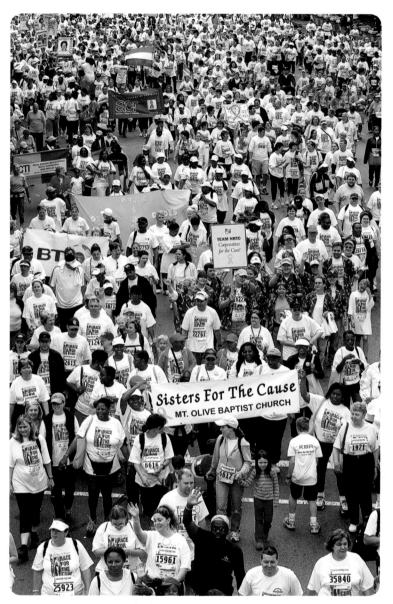

cancer—to remain dedicated to advancing research, education, screening, and treatment. We are steadfast in our faith that one day we will truly have something to celebrate: a world without breast cancer."

Afterword—Paula's Journey

"A strange and mysterious karma is working itself out in my life."

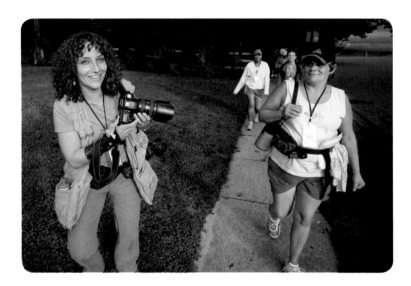

Paula Lerner has been a professional photographer for 20 years, photographing people on location for a wide variety of national and international clients. Whether it's for magazines, corporations, or institutions, says Paula, "I photograph people; I tell stories visually."

Given that much of her work over the years has focused on women's issues, *Why We Walk* was a natural fit. The fact that there was breast cancer history in her family drew her to the project on a more personal level. Both her mother and stepmother are breast cancer survivors, and in her mother's case in particular, Paula had an up-close look at the disease. "I spent a lot of time following up with doctors, being there for surgery, running interference in terms of the procedures my mother needed," says Paula, "so when Deb Murphy approached me, I was very interested in being part of the project."

Still, Paula was unprepared for what she witnessed and photographed at her first breast cancer event—the Avon Walk for Breast Cancer in Boston in May 2004. "It was unbelievably intense and moving," she recalls. "These women had incredible stories to tell about their experiences dealing with breast cancer. I was so impressed by their strength and determination and commitment." Paula also remembers looking at many of these women so close to her own age and thinking, "There but for the grace of God go I."

A month later Paula would have to reformulate that sentence to read: "A strange and mysterious karma is working itself out in my life." That June, her regular mammogram came back "suspicious." "They made me stay and speak to a radiologist," she recalls, "and I knew this was not good." A surgical biopsy was scheduled for several weeks later. In the meantime, she flew to San Francisco to cover the Avon Walk there. Compared to the event in Boston, this was a different experience. "Especially with a biopsy hanging over my head, the assignment was suddenly immediate and personal. It was no longer just something I felt strongly about. It was something I felt strongly about that was also about me."

Paula had been back in Boston for two days when they did a biopsy, and a week later she got the results. The news could have been better, but it could have been worse. She had breast cancer, but it had been detected early; she was at stage 1. Her reaction to the diagnosis was a measure of the deep connections she had forged with so many women touched by the disease. "Some women go through a 'why me?' phase. I didn't have that.

In some ways it was almost, 'Why not me?' Why does something like that happen to anybody?"

An even more pressing question, says Paula, was "What now?" Her doctors laid out the options but left the decisions regarding the course of her treatment up to her, which meant long hours of research. To determine whether or not the cancer had spread into her lymph nodes, Paula opted for a procedure called a sentinel node biopsy, or SNB. While waiting for the procedure date, she photographed the Breast Cancer 3-Day events in Washington, D.C., and Detroit.

"We began working at a little faster pace than we had anticipated," says Paula. "I wasn't sure where I was going to be in a month or two, and I felt more than ever that I wanted to finish this book because it was suddenly extremely personal." In fact, her own altered circumstances offered one appreciable advantage in her work on the project. Before she can do her job properly, she says, it's essential to make her subjects feel at ease in situations where they are likely to feel vulnerable or exposed. "When you suddenly parachute into somebody's life," as she puts it, "there is always a lag time between when they meet you and when they feel comfortable opening up to you. But after my diagnosis, that lag time was simply gone. We were all in the trenches together."

The relationship between Paula and her subjects changed in another way as well: because of her determination to push onward with the book, the women whose stories she was documenting began to look to Paula as an inspiration. "That surprised me," she says, "and I was deeply honored. The way I saw it, I was just trying to put one foot in front of the other. But having been on the other side of it not long before, I understood how just 'keeping on' can be seen as an inspiration."

Still, though, having been diagnosed with breast cancer in the middle of working on a book about the disease was "spooky and weird and just unbelievable." Working for a living is one thing; in a sense, Paula was now working for her life. "At the outset, it was a privilege to tell the stories of these women and men, but after my diagnosis it became much more than that. To be so connected to these people—to have them offer me their resources and support and love—it was a lifeline, a huge boon that I never expected."

The results from the SNB indicated that Paula's cancer was contained within her breast and had not spread to her lymph nodes. She would have to undergo a mastectomy, but was fortunate to be spared chemotherapy and radiation. She opted for a type of reconstruction surgery that "was not routine in my part of the country at that point," and for which she would have to wait more than a month. In the meantime, she photographed the Avon Walk in New York City.

The waiting, and the dread that accompanied it, seemed to have been going on all year. "In San Francisco, I was waiting to have my first biopsy. In Detroit and Washington, it was the SNB. In New York, the mastectomy lay ahead. That was hard. There was cancer in my body, and I wasn't going to start getting better until they performed that procedure, so, yeah, you bet—I did want to get it over with."

Paula's surgery took place in October, followed by a long eight weeks of recuperation. But the pathologist's report couldn't have been better. "They told me they had gotten it all—really wide margins and no further evidence of the disease." She'll be on medication for the next five years to minimize the likelihood of recurrence, but right now that likelihood is "in single digits."

"Knock wood," says Paula, "but it looks like I'm good."

Thank You All!

Finding a cure for breast cancer is the ultimate goal—thank you to all the walkers, volunteers, crew members, friends, and family who donated their time and contributed money to the cause. Know that you have made a difference and we will win this fight.

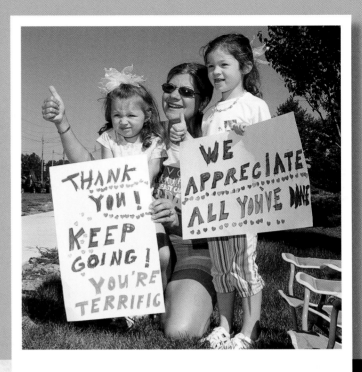

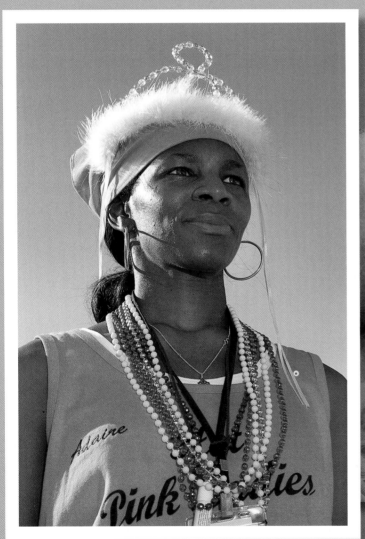

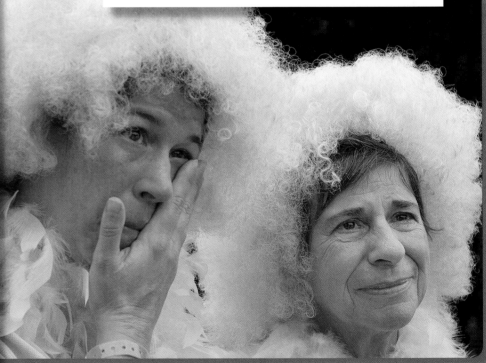

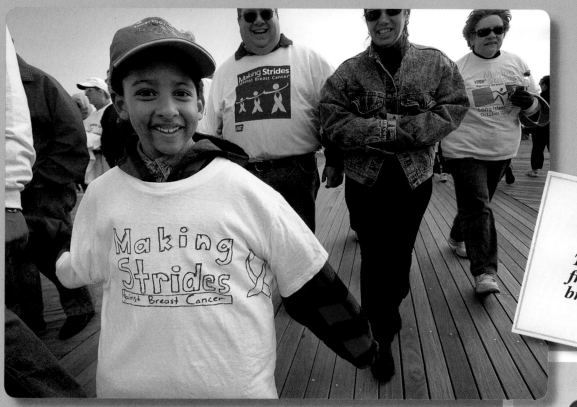

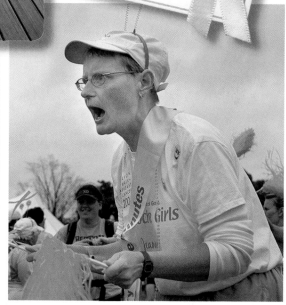

Save lives!

Talk to your
friends about
breast cancer...

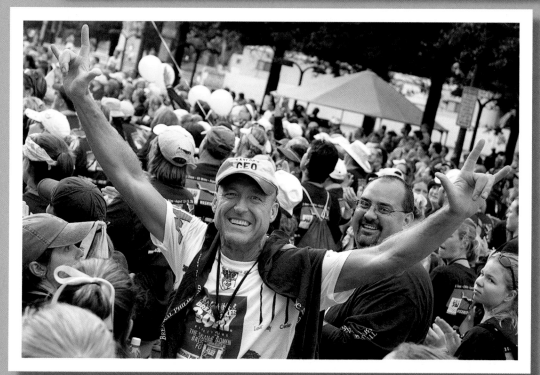

Acknowledgments

Editing this book has been an extraordinary experience and a rewarding personal journey for me, but I couldn't have done it without the help of many, many people.

First and foremost I want to thank Ralph and Shirley Wheeler, for they were my inspiration for doing the Avon Breast Cancer 3-Day in 1999. It was during those three life-changing days that I truly learned *why we walk*. I knew then that I wanted to make a book that would help others facing the challenge of breast cancer—a book that would offer the person battling cancer *encouragement* to keep fighting and offer the friends and family who were supporting this person *hope* that we will find a cure. This book is about making a difference, and every mile does make a difference.

I owe a special debt of gratitude to photographer Paula Lerner, whose personal commitment and enthusiasm for the project never waned even when she herself was diagnosed with breast cancer. Paula's photos capture the spirit and determination of the extraordinary people who participate in these events.

My special thanks to John Yow, who spent countless hours reviewing my transcripts and notes in order to write these wonderful stories. His words perfectly portray the courage and strength of the individuals we profiled.

I am enormously grateful to Lionheart Books: my business partners Michael and Lisa Reagan embraced this project and provided their ongoing support and friendship. Designer Carley Brown not only designed a beautiful book but has been a cheerleader for this project from day one. Thank you not only for your creative talent but for your many words of encouragement and enthusiasm for this project.

In addition, I would like to thank Pamela Clements at Rutledge Hill Press for believing in the book, and editor Jennifer Greenstein and copy editor Gina Webb for their thoughtful input and suggestions.

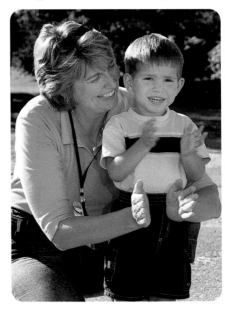

Finally, I could not have completed this book without the love and support of my friends and family: my parents, Dick and Bette Murphy; my brothers and sisters, Bob, Sue, Tom, and Laurie and their spouses and children; and of course my son, Nicholas, who is my sun, my moon, and my stars. —*Deb Murphy*

Thanks for walking!

IN CELEBRATION	IN MEMORY
Dorothy Lerner	*Nan Richter*
Mary Lerner	*Regina Roberts*
Paula Lerner	
Jean Stellrecht	
Shirley Wheeler	

Like Deb, I have found working on this book to be an extraordinary experience, especially when it became much more up close and personal than I ever imagined it might. I am thankful to all the walkers, crew, and staffers I met along the way who generously gave me the benefit of their invaluable knowledge, experience, warmth, and care.

My heartfelt thanks go to Deb Murphy for her boundless spirit, her willingness to stick with me when my cancer made things uncertain, and for tenaciously hanging in there despite a foot injury that might have sidelined others. Her drive and her good nature made collaborating a pleasure, while her good story sense and her uncanny ability to pull together the many pieces of this project have resulted in the high quality of the content here. My gratitude also goes to Carley Brown and Michael and Lisa Reagan at Lionheart Books for their commitment and contributions at every step of this endeavor from concept to completion.

Special thanks to fellow photographers Bridget Besaw Gorman and Cameron Davidson: to Bridget for pinch-hitting for me and shooting one of the walks, while I was still in the hospital, and to Cameron for taking pictures of me taking pictures at the D.C. walk after I unexpectedly became one of the stories in the book. To another fellow photographer, Rebecca Cook, my sincere gratitude for her aid as our "fixer" extraordinaire while we were covering the Komen walk in Detroit. Her work over the three-day event went above and beyond the call of duty. Hats off to Jefry Wright, Jan Schrader, Virginia Fioribello, Ghee Lip Ong, and Ana Reyes for their help as photo assistants in various cities. We couldn't have covered those walks half as well without their smiling faces and schlepping help. Additional thanks to Cathy Sachs at ASPP for originally connecting me with Deb, and to my dear friend and colleague Catherine Karnow for passing me on to Cathy.

Witnessing my mother, Dorothy Lerner, and my stepmother, Mary Lerner, survive this disease was what originally inspired me to want to do this project. I would like to thank them both, as well as my father, Bernard Lerner, my brother, Matt Lerner, and all my brothers-in-law and their respective families for their love and support when I needed it most. Lastly, I could have neither endured the difficult times after my diagnosis and treatment nor persevered to finish this book without my beloved husband, Thomas Dunlap, and our daughters, Maia and Eliana, the three of whom enabled me to keep on keeping on. —*Paula Lerner*

Special thanks to the following organizations and people who helped make this book:
Avon Walk for Breast Cancer—Karen Borkowsky, Susan Heaney, Dominick Correale
Breast Cancer 3-Day benefiting The Susan G. Komen Breast Cancer Foundation—Susan Carter, Therese Maceda, Machie Madden, Nancy Mercurio, Howard Sitron
American Cancer Society Making Strides for Breast Cancer—Michele Chiulli, Jackie Wands
National Race for the Cure—Jennifer Cawley, Kathleen Wilbur, Andy Woolard

Numerous people who volunteered their time, opened their homes, and helped us in so many different ways: Andrew Clark, Caroline Harkleroad, Anne Keiser, Doug Lapp, Ruth Krumbhaar, Linda Pruett, Jennifer Wilner

Το learn more about the organizations mentioned in this book or to make a donation, please visit their respective Web sites.

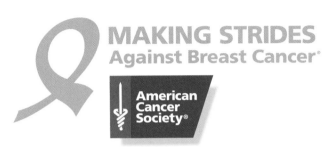

**American Cancer Society
Making Strides Against Breast Cancer**

For cancer information 24 hrs/7 days 1-800-ACS-2345
Web site: www.cancer.org
To donate and/or participate in Making Strides Against
Breast Cancer: www.cancer.org/stridesonline

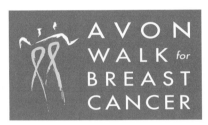

Avon Walk for Breast Cancer

c/o Avon Foundation
1345 Avenue of the Americas
New York, NY 10105
Web sites: www.avonwalk.org and www.avonfoundation.org

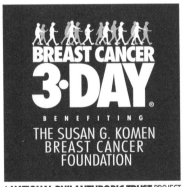

**Breast Cancer 3-Day
Benefiting the Susan G. Komen Breast Cancer Foundation**

Breast Cancer 3-Day
165 Township Line Road, Suite 150
Jenkintown, PA 19046-3594
Web site: www.the3day.org

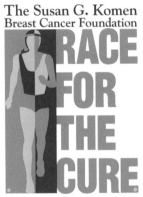

Komen Race for the Cure®

The Susan G. Komen Breast Cancer Foundation
5005 LBJ Freeway, Suite 250
Dallas, TX 75244
Toll-free Breast Care Helpline: 1-800-I'M AWARE®
(1-800-462-9273)
Web site: www.komen.org